Psychological Management of Chronic Headaches

Psychological Management of Chronic Headaches

PAUL R. MARTIN
University of Western Australia

Series Editor's Note by David H. Barlow

THE GUILFORD PRESS
New York   London

© 1993 The Guilford Press
A Division of Guilford Publications, Inc.
72 Spring Street, New York, NY 10012

Printed in the United States of America

This book is printed on acid-free paper.

Last digit is print number: 9 8 7 6 5 4 3 2

Library of Congress Cataloging-in-Publication Data

Martin, Paul R., 1951—
    Psychological management of chronic headaches / Paul R. Martin.
        p.   cm. — (Treatment manuals for practitioners)
    Includes bibliographical references and index.
    ISBN 0-89862-211-5   ISBN 1-57230-122-8 (pbk.)
    1. Headache—Psychosomatic aspects. 2. Migraine—Psychosomatic
aspects. 3. Tension headache—Psychosomatic aspects. I. Title.
II. Series.
    [DNLM: 1. Chronic Disease. 2. Headache—physiopathology.
3. Headache—psychology. 4. Headache—therapy. WL 342 M382p]
RB128.M33 1993
616.8'491—dc20
DNLM/DLC
for Library of Congress   92-48225
                                                                    CIP

For Kathryn A. Martin
and Richard C. Martin

About the Author

Paul R. Martin (D.Phil., 1977, University of Oxford) is Associate Professor of Psychology at the University of Western Australia, where he has been Director of Clinical Training and Director of the Adoption Research and Counselling Service. He maintains a clinical practice with a speciality in behavioral medicine, particularly headaches and chronic pain. Dr. Martin is a past president of the Australian Behaviour Modification Association. His most recent book is an edited volume entitled the *Handbook of Behavior Therapy and Psychological Science: An Integrative Approach*. He is on the editorial boards of *Behaviour Change* and the *International Review of Health Psychology*.

Dr. Martin has published in a number of broad areas including behavior therapy, health psychology, rehabilitation, teaching, and ethical issues, and on specific topics such as headaches, low back pain, obesity, and spasmodic torticollis. He has been involved in heachache research for many years and has received a number of grants from the National Health and Medical Research Council to support his research program. He has published extensively in the field and has given a number of keynote addresses and workshops on headaches at international conferences. Dr. Martin lives in Perth, Western Australia, with his wife and two children.

Series Editor's Note

All clinicians working with headache sufferers recognize the multi-faceted nature of these complex and difficult problems. The first generations of treatments, whether drug or non-drug, tended to be one dimensional. Headaches were broken down into broad categories and one specific treatment was prescribed based on headache type. In this book, Paul Martin, a clinician and researcher with over 15 years experience in the field of headaches, presents a second generation treatment. Based on an individualized assessment of each patient, the multiplicity of factors that research has demonstrated influence and affect headache suffering are identified and targeted for treatment. This treatment approach will "ring true" to all clinicians dealing with these problems. More importantly, the treatment is laid out in a step-by-step fashion so that clinicians dealing with headaches and related problems can readily incorporate this approach into their practice.

DAVID H. BARLOW
The University at Albany
State University of New York

Preface

This book provides a framework for conceptualizing chronic headaches. The research and psychological treatment literature relevant to this model are critically reviewed. The book then provides a detailed account of the assessment and treatment of headaches within the proposed functional framework.

The headaches that are the subject matter of this book are referred to collectively as benign recurring headaches. They include headaches diagnosed as migraine, tension headache or muscle-contraction headache (now termed *tension-type headache*), and combined or mixed headaches.

Although the book is primarily written for clinicians, it has a strong research orientation. It is hoped that it will prove useful to health professionals from a number of fields, including psychology, neurology, general/family practice, psychiatry, and other medical specialties, social work, occupational therapy, physiotherapy, and counseling.

A functional perspective has been adopted in this book. Although functional analysis occupies a central role in behavior therapy, many definitions have been offered for this approach (Haynes & O'Brien, 1990). The term has been used here to emphasize the controlling variables of headaches, or the factors that determine the variance in headache activity. The focus is on the antecedents and consequences of headaches, but these terms are defined broadly to include factors temporally remote from headaches (e.g., predisposing factors and long-term effects) as well as immediate antecedents (i.e., triggers of headaches) and immediate consequences (i.e., reactions of sufferers and significant others). Assessment of headaches is encouraged, taking into account the psychosocial and development context of headaches. Treatment is driven by the results of the functional assessment, and hence an individualized rather than a standardized approach is proposed.

The approach to treatment advocated here is similar to the cognitive–behavioral approaches described by Holroyd, Bakal, and others rather than to alternative psychological treatment approaches such as biofeedback training and relaxation training. The main point of departure, however, is that such approaches tend to equate headaches with stress whether the emphasis is on stress as a precipitant of headaches or headaches as stressors. I take the position that stress is an important factor in understanding and treating headaches but there is more to headaches than the stress–headache relationship. Headaches may be triggered by a variety of stimuli that do not fall readily into the stress category, for example, dietary factors, visual stimuli, hormonal processes, and meteorological conditions. Also, learning processes such as modeling and operant conditioning may play a role in the etiology of headaches.

I would like to acknowledge the Medical Research Council of the United Kingdom and the National Health and Medical Research Council of Australia for their contributions through the provision of research grants and scholarships in support of my headache research program. This book was planned while I was on sabbatical leave at the Center for Stress and Anxiety Disorders (State University of New York at Albany) and I am grateful to Dr. David Barlow and Dr. Edward Blanchard for the support and facilities they offered during this period. Paula Nathan worked with me in my headache research program for a number of years and I would like to thank her for her contribution toward the development of ideas and materials presented in this book. I would like to express my appreciation to my neurologist colleagues, in particular Dr. Jim Lance, Dr. Michael Anthony, and Dr. Frank Mastaglia, who supported my research, referred patients to me, and reviewed sections of this book.

I am indebted to Derek Robinson of Boehringer Ingelheim Ltd. for providing me with the three examples of "migraine art" that appear in this book. Finally, I would like to express my appreciation to Debbie McClelland for typing and retyping the manuscript.

Contents

.

Psychological Management of Chronic Headaches

1

Introduction: The Functional Model of Chronic Headaches

Most individuals have experienced a headache at one time or another, but the event is less than overwhelming and passes quite quickly. However, a significant proportion of the population experiences headaches and associated symptoms (e.g., nausea, vertigo, photophobia) of such intensity that they are quite debilitating, and many people experience headaches frequently or even continuously. Some individuals have suffered from headaches for most of their life.

The pain of the sufferer is only one aspect of the range of problems that headaches represent, however. Individuals who suffer from frequent headaches typically experience a range of associated negative emotions. Anxiety is an early response, because the sufferer worries about the cause of the headaches and the impact they will have on his or her family, social life, recreational activities, and career. If the headaches continue, other common affective reactions are frustration, anger, and confusion as the sufferer wonders why he or she is afflicted with headaches rather than someone else, and why health professionals have not cured the problem. Mild to moderate depression often sets in as headache sufferers contemplate the losses that they perceive to be caused by their headaches and begin to feel helpless and hopeless with respect to eliminating their headaches.

In addition to the emotional sequelae of headaches, headaches often result in other adverse effects, anticipated or otherwise. When headaches have spoiled social and recreational activities on a number of occasions, sufferers frequently begin to avoid such activities. This withdrawal can result in decreased physical activity/fitness, reduced social support, and loss of activities that previously provided pleasure and feelings of accomplishment. Of course, these changes often further exacerbate negative affect. Headaches can cause tension and irritability, leading to arguments at work, and severe

1

headaches can encourage absenteeism, resulting in real or imagined missed job opportunities and promotions.

Headaches affect families in many different ways. Family members share in the distress and feel helpless at their inability to prevent or abort the headaches. Partners worry about the cause of the headaches and sometimes experience anxiety and guilt over whether they are in some way responsible. Families often have to cope with a member who periodically becomes tense, sensitive, and belligerent as a result of being a headache sufferer. The withdrawal of the sufferer from social and recreational activities may result in sadness, anger, and resentment in the family.

Reactions to headaches often become problems in their own right. For example, sufferers consume large amounts of medication and then worry about the consequences to their well-being. An individual who engages in verbal or physical abuse of his or her family under the duress of headaches becomes apprehensive about the effect on family relationships, especially with children, and feels guilty for his or her actions.

Historical Overview of Psychological Research on Headaches

One would suppose that psychologists have been involved in headache research for many decades. In fact, this is not the case. Few studies were published by psychologists prior to the 1970s, which is particularly surprising since the importance of psychological factors in headaches has been recognized at least since the pioneering work of the distinguished neurologist Harold Wolff and his colleagues in the 1930s. Psychologists were largely drawn into the field as a consequence of the developing literature on biofeedback training. Headaches seemed a promising clinical application of the new technology. Since psychologists have entered the field, their research output has expanded. A bibliography of behavioral research on headaches published in 1987 included 440 papers (Martin, Marie, & Nathan, 1987). This literature is growing by approximately 50 new publications per year, and there are probably 700 papers available currently.

Psychologists, at least initially, accepted the prevailing medical models of headaches and developed treatment techniques accordingly. Hence, chronic headache sufferers were classified on the basis of their symptomatology into migraine, muscle contraction or tension headache, and mixed or combined headache types, and it was assumed that the mechanisms of migraine and tension headache were vascular and muscular, respectively. Treatment was generally aimed at regulating these physiological processes and usually involved some form of biofeedback or relaxation training. Although researchers have continued to investigate these treatment modalities, the increasing emphasis in behavior therapy on the cognitive domain has resulted in a developing literature concerned with treatment packages that include a cognitive component.

Although the initial and continuing focus of the psychological literature on headaches has been on treatment studies (P. R. Martin, 1983), some researchers began to question the traditional models on which the treatment rationales were based and consequently shifted the emphasis of their investigations. For example, the realization that the symptoms of a high proportion of headache sufferers did not closely fit the syndromes defined in the classification systems led to taxonomic research. The results of monitoring physiological processes in the laboratory led researchers to question the postulated headache mechanisms, and studies were carried out to explore the psychophysiology of headaches.

What does this now quite extensive literature have to say to the clinician? It would be nice to report that the research has clarified the nature of headaches and demonstrated that a particular approach to treatment is highly effective and superior to alternatives. Unfortunately, this is not the case. Much research has cast doubt on long-held beliefs without providing substantiated alternatives. The treatment literature has demonstrated the efficacy of a number of techniques, but none are panaceas, and it is not totally clear which are most effective or why they work. Also, the research literature is likely to seem unsatisfactory to clinicians for a number of reasons. First, the literature consists of evaluations of standardized techniques or packages rather than approaches that are individualized according to the specific presenting problem, the typical method used in clinical practice. Of course, this problem has been discussed elsewhere and is one of several that have contributed to a scientist–practitioner split (Barlow, Hayes, & Nelson, 1984). The standardized approach seems particularly problematic with headaches, however, given the variety of pathways that cause individuals to suffer from headaches. From this perspective, the available treatment techniques appear somewhat superficial and symptomatic. Second, the research literature contains few practical details and seems to focus almost exclusively on head pain rather than the associated problems discussed at the beginning of this chapter.

Although I have criticized the research literature, it should be noted that it also has much to offer clinicians. The problem is how to organize the quite extensive literature and build a viable clinical approach based on it. Subsequent chapters argue that the distinction between tension headaches and migraines is not a good starting point, since these types of headaches are not discrete entities; psychophysiological investigations have undermined the hypothesized muscular basis of tension headaches, and there is little evidence to support the treatment validity of the differential diagnosis as migraine and tension headaches show similar responses to the various psychological treatment techniques. The approach taken in this book is to adopt a functional rather than traditional symptomatological perspective of headaches.

Functional Model of Chronic Headaches

A functional approach to headaches involves understanding the controlling variables of headaches and the associated psychosocial context. The key issue is why an individual suffers from a headache at one time rather than another (i.e., exploration of the variance in headache activity) in contrast to the symptomatological approach which focuses on diagnosis based on the patient's description of his or her headache experience (sensation of pain, site of pain, preceding and accompanying sensations, etc.). A functional perspective involves investigating the antecedents and consequences of headaches, including the factors that precipitate and aggravate headaches and the reactions of sufferers and those with whom they interact regularly.

The functional model of chronic headaches is shown in Figure 1.1. It should be stressed that this model is not proposed as a formal scientific theory. It is offered more as a heuristic device; it represents a method of organizing the research literature on the one hand and guiding assessment and treatment on the other. In this way, it is hoped that the model may have some value to both clinicians and researchers. The model is outlined below and evidence pertaining to it is discussed in subsequent chapters.

The headache phenomena are in the center of the model. These include the headaches and the symptoms that sometimes precede or accompany them (e.g., sensory prodromata, nausea, vomiting, vertigo, tinnitus, photophobia, phonophobia, anorexia). Also included under headache phenomena are the psychophysiological mechanisms that underlie headaches. Traditionally, these mechanisms have been purported to be distended cranial arteries for migraine and tense pericranial muscles for tension headache, but Chapter 3 argues that the evidence points more toward both types of headaches sharing a vascular mechanism.

To the left in Figure 1.1 are four categories of antecedents arranged in a temporal sequence. The "immediate antecedents" are the stimuli that precipitate or aggravate headaches. Stimuli that have been listed as triggers include stress and negative affect (anxiety, depression, anger); perceptual stimuli such as flicker, glare, eyestrain, and noise; certain foods and fasting; seasonal and meteorological factors such as heat, high humidity, and changes in weather; and menstrual factors for females. These stimuli may operate independently or aggregate in some way.

"Setting antecedents" are the life-style or life-situation factors that make an individual more or less vulnerable to headaches at a particular point in time, and are therefore related to immediate antecedents. If headaches are

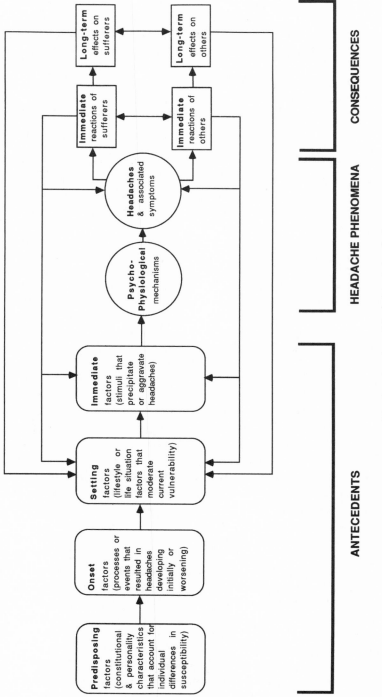

FIGURE 1.1. The functional model of chronic headaches.

ANTECEDENTS   HEADACHE PHENOMENA   CONSEQUENCES

Predisposing factors (constitutional & personality characteristics that account for individual differences in susceptibility)

Onset factors (processes or events that resulted in headaches developing initially or worsening)

Setting factors (lifestyle or life situation factors that moderate current vulnerability)

Immediate factors (stimuli that precipitate or aggravate headaches)

Psycho-Physiological mechanisms

Headaches & associated symptoms

Immediate reactions of sufferers

Immediate reactions of others

Long-term effects on sufferers

Long-term effects on others

5

precipitated by a particular stimulus, the key question from the perspective of setting factors is, Under what conditions is that stimulus most likely to occur? For example, if headaches are triggered by stress, one should search for sources of stress, as well as for factors that mediate the stress response, such as appraisal processes, coping skills, and social support systems. Setting factors are viewed as within-subject moderators of vulnerability to headaches in the sense that they can change over time.

"Onset antecedents" are the processes or events that resulted in the headache's initial development or its becoming significantly worse. Stress is often suggested as an onset factor. Head or neck trauma can lead to recurrent headaches. Hormonally mediated events may be significant for females, such as menarche, use of oral contraceptives, and pregnancy. Onset factors may or may not continue to play a significant contributory role in an individual's headache career beyond the early stages.

"Predisposing antecedents" are the constitutional and personality charac-teristics, largely determined prior to birth or in the first few years of life before headache onset, that make some individuals more likely to develop a headache problem. Headaches tend to run in families and seem to have a genetic component. Evidence suggests that some personality traits and pro-files are more common in headache sufferers than in headache-free in-dividuals; these characteristics may render an individual more liable to headaches, for example, by excessive reactions to stressful situations. Pre-disposing factors, in contrast to setting factors, are viewed as between-subject moderators of vulnerability in the sense that they are operative prior to the development of headaches and are relatively unchangeable.

Listed on the right in Figure 1.1 are the consequences of headaches divided into the immediate reactions and long-term effects for both sufferers and those with whom they interact regularly (significant others). The way sufferers and those around them react to headaches or the possibility of a headache's developing is likely to affect the experience of headaches and to have implications for the sufferer's headaches in the future. Also, the long-term impact of headaches on sufferers and their family can have implications for the sufferer's headache career.

A number of reactions to headaches are relatively maladaptive. Headaches may be maintained or increased in frequency as a result of their consequences via operant conditioning processes (reinforcement hypothesis). Thus, positive reinforcement of "headache behavior" (e.g., sympathy, atten-tion, rest) or negative reinforcement (e.g., removal of unpleasant experience or aversive situation such as missing work or avoiding interpersonal engage-ments) increases the probability of the headaches' recurrences.

Avoidance behavior may play a critical role in maintaining chronic pain (avoidance behavior hypothesis). Two variations of this hypothesis have been proposed. Philips (1987a) suggested that the short-term effect of avoidance of the stimuli that precipitate headaches is a decreased tolerance for the stimuli, and the longer-term effect is a reduction in the sufferer's belief in his or her ability to control pain. Lethem, Slade, Troup, and Bentley (1983) have proposed a fear–avoidance model of chronic pain in which they hypothesize that the individual's response when in pain (to avoid or to confront) may be instrumental in determining the chronicity of the pain or "invalid status." Fear of pain generates in some individuals a strategy of avoidance rather than confrontation, which in turn leads to both physical and psychological reinforcement of invalid status. Both versions of the avoidance behavior hypothesis clearly overlap with the reinforcement hypothesis.

Reactions to headaches and their long-term consequences can exacerbate both the immediate and setting antecedent factors (exacerbating antecedents hypothesis). This results in vicious cycles, thereby increasing headache activity. For example, headaches constitute stressors, so one possible reaction to a headache is to feel stressed. Headaches may result in family arguments, further increasing stress levels. If headaches are precipitated by stress, this completes a vicious cycle of stress–headache–stress. Taking this example further, if the arguments result in the long-term effect of marital disharmony, this may aggravate the setting factor of marital discord (as a source of stress).

Reactions to headaches may directly enhance the pain experience (enhancing pain perception hypothesis). It is well established in the pain literature that both cognitive and affective factors affect pain perception. Pain tends to be perceived more intensely than normal if the perceiver (1) focuses attention on the pain experience, (2) is anxious, and (3) does not have a sense of control over the pain. Hence, reactions to headaches and their long-term effects that involve focusing on pain, anxiety, and loss of control are likely to intensify the experience of head pain. This hypothesis overlaps the exacerbating antecedents hypothesis, since it is being suggested that headaches precipitated by stress and anxiety are likely to result in further stress and anxiety. Such reactions can be viewed as both exacerbating antecedents and enhancing pain perception directly.

Finally, a common reaction to headaches is to take medication, but there is increasing evidence that excessive consumption of ergotamine tartrate and perhaps analgesics can induce headaches (drug-induced hypothesis).

Using this model for organizing the research literature presents some problems, because it is not always clear where in the model available research data fit. For example, if headaches are associated with a particular phase of the menstrual cycle, should this be construed as an immediate or a setting factor? The answer to this question hinges on whether headaches are precipitated by menstrual cycle factors (e.g., hormonal changes) or whether such factors merely affect vulnerability to headaches, but the distinction can be subtle and may vary from one individual to another or even from one month to the next in the same subject. If the Type A coronary behavior pattern is viewed as a risk factor for headaches, does this constitute a setting or pre-disposing factor? If it is a life-style variable, which is relatively amenable to change, it would be considered a setting factor, but if it is a personality variable, which is relatively enduring, it would be considered a predisposing factor. The degree to which personality is determined by genetic versus environmental factors and the degree to which it is modifiable are issues that research has not fully resolved, thus creating uncertainty.

Also, the distinction between antecedents and consequences is often far from clear. The psychopathological abnormalities associated with headaches are usually conceptualized as causes of the head pain but could well be consequences of the pain. Many other demonstrated relationships, such as those between headaches and personality/psychopathology and between headaches and social support, leave unclear whether the identified abnormalities precede or follow the headaches.

On the other hand, perhaps one of the strengths of the model from a research perspective is the highlighting of these very issues: It is these ambiguities that need to be resolved by future studies. From a clinical perspective, some of these difficult distinctions are insignificant.

The arrows in Figure 1.1 that point from left to right reflect a temporal sequence. The bidirectional vertical arrows between the consequences of the headaches for sufferer and others are in the figure because interactions usually occur. For example, if the sufferer responds to the headaches by getting irritable and aggressive, his or her behavior usually affects the family, who often retaliate against the sufferer. The arrows between the consequences and antecedents reflect the vicious cycles that seem to occur commonly and that probably play a critical role in the etiology of chronic headaches.

Plan of the Book

This chapter briefly outlines the functional model of headaches. Part I discusses the psychological research literature pertaining to headaches. The literature review will be structured according to the functional model and research will be considered under the heading that seems currently most consistent with the data. Chapters 2 and 3 focus on headache phenomena, discussing the definition of headaches and headache types and then the psychophysiological mechanisms underlying headaches. Chapter 4 considers the antecedents and consequences of headaches, and Chapter 5 reviews the psychological treatment literature. Each review chapter concludes with a summary.

Parts II and III then discuss the practicalities of headache management. Part II focuses on the psychological assessment of headaches from a functional perspective. This part begins with a discussion of factors to consider prior to carrying out a functional analysis and is followed by a discussion of general assessment methods. Chapter 7 considers more specialized methods for assessing headache phenomena, antecedents, and consequences, and concludes with a summary of assessment methods. Two case examples of functional analysis are presented in Chapter 8.

Part III covers psychological treatment of headaches from a functional perspective. Chapter 9 develops a treatment plan based on the proposed functional assessment, treatment parameters (scheduling of sessions, treatment format, etc.), relapse prevention, and the educational component of a treatment program. Treatment strategies focusing on headache phenomena such as relaxation training, imagery training, and attention-diversion training are considered in Chapter 10. Treatment strategies focusing on the controlling variables of headaches (i.e., the antecedents and consequences) are discussed in Chapter 11. This chapter concludes with a summary of treatment methods. The final chapter describes the treatment of the two case examples presented in Chapter 8.

An example of "migraine art" is included at the beginning of each part. These illustrations convey better than words the experience that some headache sufferers have and, in particular, emphasize that headaches are often associated with a variety of distressing symptoms.

I

THE NATURE OF HEADACHES: CONCEPTUAL ISSUES AND EMPIRICAL FINDINGS

When you're lying awake with a dismal headache,
    and repose is taboo'd by anxiety,
I conceive you may use any language you choose,
    to indulge in, without impropriety.
                      —W. S. GILBERT

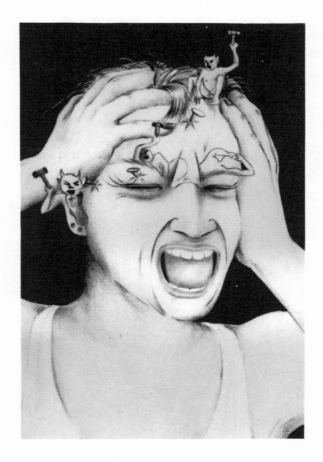

2

Headaches and
Associated Symptoms

What is a headache? The answer to this question may seem rather obvious: Dictionaries, in line with common usage, usually say something like "pain in the head" and go on to define pain as suffering, anguish, or distress (see Feuerstein, 1989, for a detailed discussion of the definition of pain). Definitions such as these immediately highlight one of the problems for practitioners, namely, that headaches refer to an experience. Headaches seem unlikely to occur in a vacuum, so one would expect a physiological substrate, associated mental activity (thoughts, images, etc.), and behavioral phenomena (coping, avoidance, etc.). However, since headaches are "private events," their investigation poses obvious problems, even though these problems are hardly unique to headaches.

Further consideration of the meaning of the term *headache* suggests that it is somewhat ambiguous and is likely to be used differently by different individuals. The ambiguities can be conceptualized as falling along two dimensions. The first is a qualitative one: Should the term be confined to pain or ache in the head or does any form of negative or unpleasant sensation in the head constitute a headache (e.g., a feeling of pressure or tenderness)? The second dimension is a quantitative one: What level of intensity or intrusiveness does an ache (or negative sensation) have to reach to constitute a headache (e.g., if the ache or unpleasant sensation was only noticed at times that attention was focused on it, would this qualify as a headache)?

Of course, it seems probable that the headaches of individuals presenting for treatment would fit the most stringent definition of the term. However, the pain thresholds and tolerances of these individuals will vary considerably, affecting the way they report their headache experience. This point was brought home dramatically when I was measuring the pain thresholds of headache sufferers and matched control subjects using a method that involves applying radiant heat to the forehead (Martin & Mathews, 1978). Some subjects reported the heat stimuli as painful at levels below my sensation threshold, while others went well past my tolerance threshold to levels that seemed in danger of causing serious burns to the skin.

Headache sufferers certainly report a wide range of headache phenomena in terms of, for example, the words they use to describe the headaches; the position of the pain; the intensity, frequency, and duration of the headaches; and the symptoms that precede, accompany, and follow the headaches. Also, all treatments (pharmacological, psychological, etc.) produce variable and unpredictable outcomes. Consequently, it is hardly surprising that researchers and clinicians have tried to categorize headache sufferers into cohesive subgroups.

Headache Classification Systems

The headache classification system that dominated the field for over a quarter of a century was formulated by a committee of six eminent neurologists in 1962 (Ad Hoc Committee, 1962). Experts in the headache field have generally considered the system outdated for some years, and consequently the International Headache Society (IHS) set up a committee to develop a revised taxonomy. This group recently published a new system, following 3 years of deliberations (Headache Classification Committee of the IHS [HCC], 1988). The older system will be outlined first, since it is this system that most headache researchers have used and most of the data relevant to classification issues pertain to this system.

The Ad Hoc Committee divided headaches into 15 major categories. The system was purportedly based on pain mechanisms, although diagnosis would often be derived from reported symptoms without direct investigation of mechanisms. The first three categories are the most common types of headaches and the ones that are the focus of this book. They consist of the following.

1. *Vascular headaches of the migraine type.* Recurrent attacks of headache, widely varied in intensity, frequency and duration. The attacks are commonly unilateral in onset, are usually associated with anorexia and sometimes with nausea and vomiting; in some are preceded by, or associated with, conspicuous sensory, motor, and mood disturbances; and often familial. Evidence supports the view that cranial arterial distention and dilatation are importantly implicated in the pain phase, but cause no permanent changes in the involved vessel (Ad Hoc Committee, 1962, p. 717). Five subtypes are then listed: classic migraine, common migraine, cluster headache, hemiplegic or opthalmoplegic migraine, and lower half headache.

2. *Muscle-contraction headache*. Ache or sensations of tightness, pressure, or constriction, widely varied in intensity, frequency, and duration, sometimes long-lasting and commonly suboccipital. It is associated with sustained contraction of skeletal muscles in the absence of permanent structural change, usually as part of the individual's reaction during life stress. The ambiguous and unsatisfactory terms "tension", "psychogenic", and "nervous" headache refer largely to this group (Ad Hoc Committee, 1962, p. 717).

3. *Combined headache: Vascular and muscle-contraction.* Combinations of vascular headache of the migraine type and muscle-contraction headache, prominently coexisting in an attack (Ad Hoc Committee, 1962, p. 717).

This classification system was lacking in detail as illustrated by the fact that the descriptions include all the information in the system about these three categories of headaches with the exception that each of the migraine subtypes was described briefly. Reflecting modern trends in taxonomies, the IHS system includes operational diagnostic criteria for all types of headaches, resulting in a system that is described in a special supplement of the society's journal *Cephalalgia* and spans 96 pages (in contrast to the 2 pages of the Ad Hoc Committee's system). The strengths and weaknesses of the old and new systems have been reviewed recently by Rapoport (1992).

The IHS system divides headaches into 13 major categories, the first two of which are migraine and tension-type headache. The 13 major categories, and the subcategories of migraine and tension-type headache, appear in Appendix 1. Descriptions of the two main subcategories of migraine and the three subcategories of tension-type headache are included in Appendix 2.

The term *combined headache* (or equivalent) does not appear in the IHS system, but patients may suffer from more than one type of headache (headaches are classified, not patients). Cluster headache appears as a separate headache category rather than a subtype of migraine. Seven subcategories of migraine are listed, some of which are further subdivided. The terms *classic migraine* and *common migraine* have been dropped because they convey no information, and they have been replaced by *migraine with aura* and *migraine without aura*, the aura being the complex of focal neurological symptoms that initiates or accompanies an attack.

The term *tension-type headache* has been used to cover headaches previously referred to as tension headache, muscle-contraction headache, and psychogenic headache. This category is now subdivided into four main subcategories. Tension-type headaches are grouped as "episodic" or "chronic" depending on their frequency. This distinction was introduced because patients with daily or almost daily headaches constitute a large group in specialized practices and hospital clinics. Each of these subcategories is then further subdivided on the basis of whether the headache is or is not associated with disorder of pericranial muscles. This novel distinction has been added due to controversy over whether tension headaches are indeed caused by skeletal muscle tension. The evidence surrounding this controversy will be reviewed in Chapter 3. It is noted in the classification system that the mechanism of "tension-type headache unassociated with disorder of pericranial muscles [is unknown,] but psychogenic etiologies are suspected" (HCC, 1988, p. 31).

Although the two systems discussed above are the most important ones focusing on headaches, two others will be discussed briefly. The International Association for the Study of Pain (IASP) has recently prepared the first "Classification of Chronic Pain" (Merskey, 1986). It is a multiaxial system with five axes: regions, systems, temporal characteristics of pain and pattern of occurrence, patient's statement of intensity and time since onset of pain, and etiology. "Acute tension headache" and "tension headache: chronic form" are listed under "Craniofacial Pain of Musculoskeletal Origin" (p. S58), but it is noted that "vessels or central nervous system" are involved "according to some opinions". "Classical migraine", "common migraine", "migraine variants", "mixed headache", and "cluster headache", are categorized as "Primary Headache Syndromes" (pp. S71–S74), and it is suggested that the system responsible for migraine is unknown but "vascular disturbances have been emphasized" and "central nervous system changes may be fundamental."

Finally, it is important to note the place of headaches in the International Classification of Diseases (ICD-IX) (World Health Organization [WHO], 1977) given that this latter system is the official taxonomy of the World Health Organization and is in widespread use internationally. The term *migraine* appears under "other disorders of the central nervous system" (WHO, 1977, p. 227) in Section VI, Diseases of the Nervous System and Sense Organs. On the other hand, tension headaches are included under "neurotic disorders, personality disorders and other nonpsychotic mental disorders" (WHO, 1977, p. 204) in Section V, Mental Disorders. Tension headaches, along with psychogenic backache, are viewed as forms of "psychalgia" defined as "cases in which there are pains of mental origin where a more precise medical or psychiatric diagnosis cannot be made" (WHO, 1977, p. 204). Consideration of how tension headache fits into ICD-IX reveals how a segment of the medical profession views this type of headache and may explain why headache sufferers often seek the label *migraine* rather than *tension headache*.

Evaluation of Headache Classification Systems

From an empirical perspective, a number of questions can be generated with respect to the symptomatology of chronic headaches. Are the data (i.e., symptoms) best described by a categorical or a dimensional model, and how many categories or dimensions should such a model include? The classification systems, of course, are based on a categorical approach and define two major types. Migraine and tension headache are viewed as discrete entities, although it is noted in the IHS system that the separation of migraine without aura from episodic tension-type headache may be difficult. Before trying to answer these difficult questions, a simpler one should be considered. Can tension headaches and mirgraines be differentiated reliably? This question makes no assumptions about categorical versus dimensional models or whether the syndromes described in the classification system are necessarily the optimal groupings of symptoms.

The evidence pertaining to differential diagnosis seems to indicate that quite satisfactory levels of reliability can be achieved. Turkat, Brantley, Orton, and Adams (1981) reported agreement ranging from 62% to 64% among three doctoral clinical psychology students diagnosing headaches. Somewhat higher agreement was reported in two subsequent studies, with Blanchard, O'Keefe, Neff, Jurish, and Andrasik (1981) finding agreement in 81% of cases between a neurologist and clinical psychologist and Drummond and Lance (1984) obtaining agreement between a neurologist and a computer classification procedure in 90% of cases. It seems reasonable to predict that even greater reliability will be attained with the IHS classification system given its emphasis on operational criteria.

The evidence is more mixed and complex with respect to the issue of syndromes. In a large epidemiological study, Waters (1973) found little evidence that three features considered characteristic of migraine (a unilateral distribution, a warning that a headache is coming, and nausea accompanying a headache) occurred in the same individual more frequently than would be expected on the basis of chance occurrences depending simply on the separate prevalences of each feature. He did report that with each of the three features, the prevalence increased with the severity of the headache. In the first factor-analytic study of headache symptoms, Ziegler, Hassanein, and Hassanein (1972) analyzed questionnaire data elicited from a series of 289 consecutive patients seeking help for headaches. They found that migraine features were distributed among three factors, and that some features usually considered indicative of migraine were not associated with any of these three. One factor was suggestive of tension headaches, but again features usually linked with tension headaches were not correlated with this factor.

Using a methodology different from the one in the above studies, Bakal and Kaganov (1977) divided 56 headache sufferers into the first three categories of the Ad Hoc Committee's classification using neurologists' diagnoses. Subjects were then asked to self-monitor headache symptoms over a 2-week period. The results suggested that migraine and tension headache sufferers had similar symptoms (e.g., no difference between the groups in percentage of who had throbbing headache, associated visual disturbances, or a family history of headaches, but significantly more migraine patients suffered from nausea and vomiting). The results of this study and others by this group of workers (e.g., Joffe, Bakal, & Kaganov, 1983) has led Bakal to propose a psychobiological or severity model of headaches in which he argues that headache patients differ from occasional sufferers as well as from each other primarily in terms of the frequency with which the various symptoms are experienced and not in terms of the types of symptoms experienced (Bakal & Kaganov, 1979).

Peck and Attfield (1981) replicated the finding of Ziegler et al. (1972) that no factor emerged that combined the variables ordinarily thought of as particularly characteristic of migraine, but their results were not consistent with Waters's suggestion that headache severity correlated with the presence of three migraine features. Drummond and Lance (1984), in the study referred to earlier, failed to obtain a clear distinction between migraine and tension headache and found that patients described a broad spectrum of symptoms progressively declining from severe, episodic headaches associated with many migraine features to constant headaches with few or no migraine features.

In contrast to the above studies, Arena, Blanchard, Andrasik, and Dudek (1982) argued that the results of their factor-analytic investigation lent support to there being two global headache categories corresponding to migraine and tension headache. Also, Mindell and Andrasik (1987) found a similar result with children who suffered from headaches. In a recent study, Takeshima and Takahashi (1988) carried out a number of multivariate analyses on headache symptoms. A tension headache and migraine factor emerged from a principal-components analysis, but the authors interpreted their findings as contrary to the concept of tension headaches and migraines as separate entities. They argued for these two types of headaches lying at the extremes of a continuum but partly disagreed with the headache severity model because their data indicated that there were qualitative rather than quantitative differences between the two types of headaches. The revised severity model proposed by Takeshima and Takahashi consists of a continuum but with two dimensions, corresponding to the migraine factor and the tension headache factor, rather than one.

Iversen, Langemark, Andersson, Hansen, and Olesen (1990) reported an early study of the IHS classification system. Their main result was that the new operational criteria of this system did not radically change the diagnosis of patients with migraine or tension headache.

I have suggested elsewhere that a more radical departure from the old classification may be necessary than those discussed above (Martin, 1985). An argument was developed in Chapter 1 for adopting a functional rather than a symptomatological approach. In my research, I have explored whether categorical or dimensional models can be developed based on functional characteristics of headaches (i.e., controlling variables) rather than headache symptoms (Martin, Milech, & Nathan, 1992). Using cluster analysis, we found that headache sufferers could not be categorized into cohesive subgroups on the basis of functional characteristics. Factor-analyzing antecedents and consequences resulted in a number of interpretable factors emerging, however. The immediate antecedents of headaches yielded five dimensions, immediate responses of sufferers yielded three dimensions, and immediate reactions of others yielded three dimensions. A preliminary analysis showed that some antecedent and consequences dimensions were better predictors of response to psychological treatment than were traditional diagnostic categories. The antecedent and consequences dimensions are discussed in Chapter 4 and their predictive significance is discussed in Chapter 5.

Prevalence of Headaches

Most individuals are familiar with the experience of a headache and frequent headaches are a common problem. Making more precise statements presents difficulties, however, as epidemiological studies have reported prevalence figures that vary considerably. The distinguished British epidemiologist Waters suggested that the explanation of conflicting findings on the prevalence of migraine, probably lay in methodological differences among the various surveys and differences in the diagnostic criteria for migraine rather than in real differences in prevalence between populations (Waters, 1978). Whereas methodological differences and diagnostic criteria seem almost certain to play a role in discrepant findings, real differences may also explain some of the variance. An example of the latter possibility comes from my own work. We carried out a survey of the prevalence of headaches in Australian university students (Martin & Nathan, 1987). We instigated this study because we were surprised to read of the high prevalence of headaches in North American college students. Andrasik, Holroyd, and Abell (1979) reported that 52.7% of such students suffered from one to two headaches per week or more, and 20% suffered from three to four headaches per week or more. Using their questionnaire on an equivalent population (first-year undergraduate psychology students), we found that only 20.4% of Australian students suffered from one to two headaches per week or more and only 5.5% suffered from three to four headaches per week or more. We suggested that the explanation for these large differences in prevalence (i.e., factors of 2.6 and 3.6 for the two cumulative frequencies) lay in differences in stressors and factors that mediate the stress response (Martin & Nathan, 1987). The important point here, however, is that these data emphasize the need for great caution in extrapolating findings from one population to another even when the populations appear highly similar.

Headaches, including migraine, have been diagnosed in children as young as 18 months (Selby & Lance, 1960). Sillanpaa (1976) carried out a study of headaches in 7-year-old children in Finland and found that 37.7% had headaches before starting school. In his sample, 6.7% experienced headaches once a week or more frequently, and he suggested that 3.2% of the sample suffered from migraine. The prevalence of headaches seems to increase through childhood and adolescence. Sillanpaa (1983), for example, followed up the children from his earlier study when they reached age 14 and reported that 69% had experienced headaches by this age. He found that 9% suffered headaches once a week or more frequently and 10.6% of the sample were migraineurs. Similar patterns of increasing childhood headache prevalence with age have been reported in other studies (e.g., Bille, 1962).

Although childhood headaches were once viewed as a transient phenomenon which the child would outgrow (Ryan, 1954), there is increasing evidence from longitudinal studies to suggest that this is not so. Bille (1981), for instance, found that 60% of children between ages 7 and 15 who were diagnosed as suffering from migraine continued to report symptoms into adulthood. On the other hand, early childhood is an uncommon time for headache onset compared to later periods. Epidemiological studies show that headache problems most commonly begin in the second, third, or fourth decades of life; this 30-year span accounts for 80% to 90% of headache onsets (Levy, 1983; Phanthumchinda & Sithi-Amorn, 1989; Zhao et al., 1988).

With respect to adult samples, Ziegler, Hassanein, and Couch (1977), in a study of the general population in the United States, found an overall headache prevalence of 83%, with 47.6% suffering from severe or disabling headaches. Lower figures have been reported from other developed countries. Nikiforow and Hokkanen (1978), for example, found a prevalence of 65.8% in Finland, and Paulin, Waal-Manning, Simpson, and Knight (1985) reported a prevalence of 49.9% in New Zealand. Prevalence in less developed countries is more variable, with Sachs et al. (1985) arguing that their data from a rural village in Ecuador were remarkably similar to data reported from the United States and Europe but Levy (1983) reporting an overall headache prevalence of only 20.2% in her study of an urban population in Zimbabwe.

These studies consistently report sex differences, with headaches being more common in females than in males. In the study by Nikiforow and Hokkanen (1978), for example, the prevalence rates were 73.1% for women and 57.6% for men. Nikiforow and Hokkanen reported that education, social class, and mode of employment did not influence the prevalence of headaches.

With respect to the frequency of headaches, Nikiforow and Hokkanen

(1978) found that 24.3% of their total sample suffered from mild headaches once a week or more, while 9.9% suffered from severe headaches once a week or more. These findings are similar to those reported by Waters (1974), who recorded 20% of a Welsh sample as experiencing one or more headaches per week. In Waters's study, the most commonly reported average headache duration was 1 to 4 hours, with few respondents indicating an average duration of over 12 hours.

Attempts at establishing the prevalence rates of specific headache types have produced wildly discrepant results. In a critical review of headache prevalence in male samples, for example, Ekbom, Ahlborg, and Schele (1978) tabulated rates varying from 1.5% to 26.1% for migraine and 2.6% to 65.5% for "nonmigrainous" headaches. The research showed only that tension headaches seem more common than migraines and cluster headaches are comparatively rare.

Estimates of the number of headache sufferers in the United Kingdom and the United States who consult a doctor range from 10% to 50% (Newland, Illis, Robinson, Batchelor, & Waters, 1978; Andrasik et al., 1979). One important implication of this low attendance rate is that clinic samples of headache patients are not necessarily representative of headache sufferers in the general population. There is no doubt that clinic samples are unrepresentative in some ways such as sex distribution. DeLozier and Gagnon (1975) reported, for example, that among individuals seeking outpatient medical care for headaches in the United States, females outnumbered males 2.4 to 1 in contrast to the marginally higher population prevalence rates in females described above. Most headache research studies include two to three times as many female subjects as male subjects.

Finally, with respect to headache prevalence, a number of studies have documented a significant decline in incidence in later life (Nikiforow & Hokkanen, 1978; Waters, 1974).

Summary

All the major headache classification systems include the categories of tension headache and migraine, although different terms have often been used. The systems differ with respect to whether cluster headache is included as a type of migraine or as a separate entity (the trend is toward the latter), whether combined or mixed headaches are included (the IASP classification includes the category but suggests that the term should probably be abandoned), the subcategories of the main two types, and the hypothesized pain mechanisms. In this book the terms *tension headache* and *migraine* will be used rather than the alternatives.

The results of factor-analytic studies of headache symptoms are mixed—

some support migraine and tension headache syndromes and some do not. The majority of researchers argue against migraine and tension headache as discrete entities and instead favor conceptualizing them as opposite ends of a spectrum, continuum, or dimension (e.g., Waters, 1973; Bakal & Kaganov, 1979; Philips, 1977a; Takeshima & Takahashi, 1988). The most popular view is that the continuum is a single dimension that corresponds to headache severity (migraine at the more extreme pole), but some have argued for modification of this severity model. It is interesting to note that this conceptualization contrasts with the one underlying the Ad Hoc Committee's classification and also the new IHS and IASP systems. I have argued for conceptualizing chronic headaches on the basis of functional characteristics rather than symptoms and have developed a dimensional model driven by controlling variables (Martin, 1985; Martin, Milech, & Nathan, 1992).

Headaches are a common problem. Their reported prevalence rates generally range from 66% to 83% in developed countries. The prevalence of headaches increases through childhood and stabilizes in adult life prior to decreasing during old age. Headaches are more common in females than in males, but their prevalence is unrelated to variables such as education, social class, and type of employment. Only 10–50% of headache sufferers consult physicians.

3

Psychophysiological
Mechanisms of Headaches

As mentioned in Chapter 2, the Ad Hoc Committee's classification proposed separate, peripheral pain mechanisms for tension headaches and migraines: The former were considered "associated with sustained contraction of skeletal muscles" and the latter "associated with cranial arterial distention and dilatation" (Ad Hoc Committee, 1962, p. 717). Essentially, the rationales for psychological treatments have been based on these hypothesized mechanisms, and psychophysiologically orientated headache research has focused mainly on muscular and cardiovascular variables. Hence, these psychophysiological mechanisms are discussed here. It should be noted, however, that other mechanisms have been proposed for benign recurring headaches, particularly migraine. In the IHS system, for example, tension headaches are still considered caused by muscle tension or factors unknown, but a number of possible mechanisms are listed for migraine, including changes in regional cerebral blood flow, changes in blood composition and platelet function initiated endogenously or by environmental influences, and pathophysiological processes in the brain that, via the trigemino-vascular and other systems, interact with intra- and extracranial vasculature and perivascular spaces (HCC, 1988). Saper (1989) lists eight theories of migraine and notes that in recent years, a number of leading physicians in the field have switched their attention from peripheral to central mechanisms. However, review of these theories is beyond the scope of this book.

Another area to consider before discussing the evidence relating to psychophysiological mechanisms is measurement issues. Assessing muscular hypotheses by measuring electromyographic (EMG) activity presents relatively few technical or interpretive problems. Perhaps one minor exception relates to whether it is possible to generalize from one muscle site to others. Some researchers have implied that generalization is acceptable by, for example,

23

suggesting that forehead EMG biofeedback training is a general relaxation technique, but such inferences are probably not warranted (Alexander, 1975).

In contrast, investigating vascular hypotheses is fraught with difficulties. The most common approach has been to measure the state of dilation of arteries indirectly via photoplethysmography, which is based on the principle that light reflected from the tissue under the transducer is a function of local blood flow (Jennings, Tahmoush, & Redmond, 1980). A host of factors other than blood flow may affect the signal recorded by the polygraph, however, such as the precise position of the transducer relative to the artery, how the transducer is attached to the skin, skin characteristics, and technical parameters of the recording apparatus. Researchers have responded to these problems by using relative rather than absolute measures in their analyses (Haynes, Cuevas, & Gannon, 1982). Pulse amplitude is used as the unit of measurement, for example, which consists of the amount of displacement in the polygraph signal caused by the passage of the pressure pulse along the artery. Also, some researchers analyze changes in pulse amplitude from baseline recordings rather than absolute pulse amplitudes.

Some experts on plethysmography have argued that a consequence of the methodology's being an indirect measure, and one that is affected by a number of variables, is that plethysmography results cannot be compared between laboratories, individuals, or even the same individuals on different occasions (Jennings et al., 1980). If this argument is accepted, the approach has serious limitations for investigating headache mechanisms, because most vascular hypotheses pertain to differences between headache sufferers and nonheadache controls, or between individuals when suffering from a headache and when headache free. Also, using pulse amplitude as the unit of measurement results in a confounding of two variables: distension of the artery between pressure pulses and distension of the artery during the passage of pressure pulses. The relationship between arterial diameter and pulse amplitude depends on when distension occurs: Distension during the passage of the pulse but not between pulses would result in an increase in pulse amplitude, equal distension during and between pulses would result in no change in pulse amplitude, and distension between pulses but not during passage of the pulses would result in a decrease in pulse amplitude.

Another problem with the approach commonly used is that it provides no information about mechanisms of change in vascular activity. Headache researchers have frequently interpreted observed changes in pulse amplitude as indicating peripheral sympathetic vasomotor activity. Such an inference is not justified because observed changes may arise from alterations elsewhere in the cardiovascular system (e.g., blood pressure and heart rate). Put simply, an artery may be distended as a result of relaxation of local smooth muscle or elevated blood pressure. For this reason, experts in the measurement of peripheral vascular activity recommend that other cardiovascular variables should also be measured (Jennings et al., 1980).

Tension Headache

Skeletal Muscle Activity

Researchers investigating the muscular activity associated with tension headaches have addressed a number of different hypotheses: (1) tension headaches arise from generally elevated levels of muscle tension (i.e., tension is high regardless of whether the individual is suffering from a headache or not); (2) tension headaches result from an excessive increase in tension levels in responses to stress; (3) tension headaches arise from a slow recovery of tension levels following stress; and (4) tension headache sufferers have a low threshold for pain from muscle tension. Often three or all four of these hypotheses have been addressed in a single study. In one of my early studies we compared the forehead and neck EMG levels of tension headache sufferers and individually matched controls in response to the three experimental conditions of rest, stress (speeded problem-solving), and poststress recovery (Martin & Mathews, 1978). The two groups did not significantly differ on either measure of muscle tension under any of the three conditions. This result was quite unexpected at the time, so the data were reanalyzed in various ways to try to unearth the missing muscle tension. In one analysis, data were included only for headache sufferers experiencing a headache at the time of recording and their corresponding controls. This change did not alter the pattern of nonsignificant findings. The data were also reanalyzed excluding all but the most clear-cut cases of tension headaches, to protect against the possibility of including diagnostically inappropriate cases. Again, this did not affect the findings.

Many other studies have used a similar experimental paradigm but with different stressors (e.g., mental arithmetic, stressful imagery, noise stimuli, cold pressor) and recording from different muscle sites (e.g., temporalis, trapezius, occipitalis). The results of such studies are mixed, with each of the muscular hypotheses supported by some findings but not by others. Flor and Turk (1989) recently reviewed these studies and concluded that there is limited evidence to support the notion of permanently elevated EMG levels in tension headache sufferers. They made the interesting observation that among studies they rated as more methodologically sound, compared to studies that were methodologically weaker, a lower proportion reported positive findings (i.e., supported the muscular hypothesis).

Flor and Turk (1989) argued that there is more support for EMG reactivity to stress as a headache mechanism, a conclusion similar to one I reached in an earlier review of the literature (Martin, 1986). One line of reasoning in support of this conclusion is that it is easier to explain away nonsignificant findings for reactivity data than for resting levels data: Researchers who have failed to find significant differences may have used stressors that are not sufficiently potent for individual subjects or prolonged. Inspection of much of the data seems consistent with the possibility that significant findings emerge when more aversive stressors are used. Contrast, for example, the 6-minute stress condition in our study (Martin & Mathews, 1978) with the 25-minute stress condition (Cohen, Williamson, et al., 1983) that apparently led many subjects to complain that it was too taxing. The latter study reported significant findings in contrast to the former study. On the other hand, a recent study by Gannon, Haynes, Cuevas, and Chavez (1987) used a 60-minute stressor and found no significant differences in EMG reactivity between tension headache sufferers and controls, so the issue is still far from clear. The review by Flor and Turk (1989) is potentially misleading with respect to EMG reactivity to stress because they include studies of both reactivity to pain and reactivity to stress. Hence, studies that have found higher EMG levels for headache sufferers experiencing a headache than for control subjects are counted as supporting the reactivity hypothesis. Although head pain can clearly be viewed as a stressor, positive findings from such studies can reflect muscle tension as a consequence rather than a cause of headaches.

With respect to the poststress recovery hypothesis, Flor and Turk (1989), reporting approximately equal numbers of positive and negative findings, found the evidence inconclusive. Flor and Turk only included studies that directly tested this hypothesis, however, rather than others that tested it indirectly (e.g., Martin & Mathews, 1978). When these other studies are taken into account, the supportive evidence at present seems very thin.

Turning to the threshold hypothesis, early studies did not support lower pain thresholds in terms of heat stimuli applied to the head (Martin & Mathews, 1978) or pressure stimuli applied to the fingers (Feuerstein, Bush, & Corbisiero, 1982). On the other hand, Borgeat, Hade, Elie, and Larouche (1984) demonstrated lower pain thresholds in tension headache sufferers compared with controls to pain induced by tensing forehead muscles. Drummond (1987) measured pressure–pain thresholds at six head and neck locations of tension headache sufferers and controls and found that the headache subjects had significantly lower thresholds during headaches and within 5 days of a headache, but the difference had disappeared at more than 5 days after the headache. A recent study by Schoenen, Bottin, Hardy, and Gerard (1991) found that individual values for pressure–pain thresholds were widely scattered but were, on average, significantly lower in tension headache sufferers than in controls. Hence, studies on pain thresholds suggest that tension headache sufferers do not have a generally lower pain threshold across pain stimuli and body location but do have a lower threshold for certain types of pain stimuli (e.g., pressure, tension) in the region of the head at least during or within a few days of a headache.

Studies considered so far have analyzed between-subjects data. Other evidence relevant to muscular mechanisms comes from within-subjects analyses. Several studies have compared EMG data between headache and headache-free periods with mixed results. For example, Haynes, Griffin, Mooney, and Parise (1975) found significantly higher forehead EMG levels during headache periods, Martin and Mathews (1978) reported the reverse (significantly lower forehead EMG during headaches), and no significant difference in neck EMG, and Philips (1977b) found no significant differences in forehead, neck, trapezius, or temporalis EMG. The conflicting results of these early studies have continued into the recent literature, with some studies reporting elevated EMG in headache compared to nonheadache states (e.g., Murphy & Lehrer, 1990) and other studies reporting no significant differences (e.g., Martin, Marie, & Nathan, 1992; Lichstein et al., 1991). Martin and Mathews (1978) calculated correlation coefficients between headache intensity and simultaneously recorded forehead and neck EMG. Averaging these correlations across the sample resulted in a correlation of $r = -.10$ between headache intensity and forehead EMG, and $r = .02$ between headache intensity and neck EMG.

The rationale for providing EMG biofeedback training to tension headache sufferers was to teach them to reduce or eliminate the muscle tension causing the headaches, and studies that demonstrated concurrent decreases in headache activity and EMG levels were sometimes cited as evidence supporting a muscular mechanism. As the EMG biofeedback literature has developed, however, the findings have cast further doubt on muscular hypotheses rather than bolstering them. For example, a number of researchers have calculated correlation coefficients between decreases in forehead EMG and tension headaches and found them to be nonsignificant (e.g., Holroyd & Andrasik, 1978; Holroyd, Andrasik, & Westbrook, 1977; Martin & Mathews, 1978). Even more persuasive are data from a study by Andrasik and Holroyd (1980a) in which three biofeedback conditions and a no-treatment procedure were compared. All biofeedback groups were instructed similarly and were led to believe that they were learning to reduce forehead EMG activity. In fact, training focused on teaching subjects to decrease, increase, or hold stable forehead EMG activity. Results indicated that while EMG activity shifted in the intended direction, the headaches of the three biofeedback groups all improved significantly and equally.

Other Psychophysiological Mechanisms

Because traditional views of tension headaches have involved muscular mechanisms, other physiological variables have not been investigated extensively or systematically. Some studies have measured such variables as temporal and digital blood flow, hand temperature, heart rate, systolic and diastolic blood pressure, respiration rate, and skin resistance. A number of positive findings have been reported pertaining to various vascular measures. Ahles et al. (1988) reported the curious finding of what they interpreted as vasoconstriction in the left temporal artery but not in the right in tension headache sufferers relative to controls during recording of subjects in a number of different postures (reclining, sitting, and standing). Bakal and Kaganov (1977) found a decrease in blood flow velocity recorded from the right and left temporal arteries in response to noise in tension headache sufferers but the opposite response in controls. No EMG abnormalities were found in a study by Lehrer and Murphy (1991), but these researchers reported higher heart rate and evidence of more prolonged vasoconstriction in the hands and the earlobes of tension headache sufferers relative to controls.

Haynes and Gannon and their colleagues have reported a number of findings of relevance here. In one study, they observed that the heart rates of tension headache subjects who reported a headache during a stressor were significantly higher than the heart rates of controls (Gannon et al., 1987). Haynes et al. (1983) recorded blood volume pulse (BVP) from the left earlobe during headache-free and headache periods and reported that six subjects demonstrated significantly greater vasoconstriction in the headache period, one subject demonstrated significantly greater vasodilation in the headache period, and no significant differences between periods were found for two subjects. In a recent study, this group found significant correlations between induced headache reports in a predominantly tension headache sample and cephalic BVP amplitude measures for most subjects (Haynes, Gannon, Bank, Shelton, & Goodwin, 1990).

In two of my studies that have failed to find EMG abnormalities associated with tension headaches, vascular abnormalities have been demonstrated. An early study included administering amyl nitrite, a potent vasodilating agent, and a placebo in a counterbalanced order to a series of tension headache subjects and asking them to rate their headache intensity before and after inhaling each drug (Martin & Mathews, 1978). Inhaling amyl nitrite led to an increase in reported head pain in 43% of patients tested compared with only one patient's reporting a decrease in pain. No patient reported an increase in pain following inhaling the placebo, suggesting that tension headaches are associated with vasodilation at least for some subjects. In a more recent study, we attempted to overcome the vascular hypothesis measurement problems discussed at the beginning of this chapter (Martin,

Marie, & Nathan, 1992). Specifically, we measured maximum, minimum, and average distension of the superficial temporal artery, and rather than calculating difference scores between the maximum and minimum values, which would approximate the usual pulse amplitude measure, the measures were analyzed separately to avoid confounding. We also included continuous measures of blood pressure and heart rate so that the mechanisms of vascular changes could be explored. Tension headache sufferers and controls were compared across four experimental conditions: rest, pain induction, recovery, and pain reduction.

We found that tension headache subjects compared to controls had distended superficial temporal arteries between pressure pulses, but not during the passage of pressure pulses, and had elevated blood pressure across conditions. Further analysis suggested that local vasomotor activity might play a role in dilating the temporal artery but that the effect seemed driven by elevated blood pressure and heart rate.

Hence, a number of studies have provided evidence suggesting that tension headaches are associated with some form of vascular dysfunction. It must be emphasized, however, that other studies have monitored vascular variables from headache sufferers and controls and not reported significant findings. In fact, a number of studies have measured multiple variables and failed to find significant results for any of them (e.g., Anderson & Franks, 1981; Andrasik, Blanchard, Arena, Saunders, & Barron, 1982; Feuerstein et al., 1982). Drawing conclusions from the literature is further hampered by the complexity of the cardiovascular system and consequent difficulties in interpreting the meaning of cardiovascular findings. Bakal and Kaganov (1977), for example, interpreted a decrease in pulse velocity as indicating vasoconstriction. Pulse velocity is a product of both state of distension of an artery and blood pressure, so it is not possible to infer one variable from knowledge of only one other variable; however, even if it was assumed that blood pressure remained constant (a dubious assumption given its lability), a decrease in velocity would seem to suggest vasodilation rather than vasoconstriction.

Migraine

Cardiovascular Activity

The classic model of migraine is a two-stage process, with intra- and extracranial vasoconstriction during the preheadache or prodromal phase (O'Brien, 1971; Ostfeld & Wolff, 1958) followed by a rebound phenomenon of intra- and extracranial vasodilation during the headache phase (Dalessio, 1972; Tunis & Wolff, 1953). The vasoconstriction can produce ischemia, and sensory prodromata, such as visual disturbances, may result (Skinhoj & Paulson, 1969). At the onset of headache, pulsatory head pain results from the increased amplitude of the extracranial vasculature, which in turn distends surrounding pain-sensitive fibers. As the attack progresses, the pain becomes steady rather than pulsatory, and concurrently, a sterile inflammation and edema are produced in the extracranial arteries, rendering them thickened and rigidified (Dalessio, 1972, 1974). This two-stage model evolved out of early experiments that manipulated the extracranial vasomotor activity of the temporal artery via administration of ergotamine tartrate (a vasoconstrictive substance) and finger pressure over the artery (e.g., Graham & Wolff, 1938). These studies showed a close relationship between vasomotor activity and reported head pain.

It has often been argued that stress can lead to a migraine attack by triggering temporal vasoconstriction followed by a rebound vasodilation. This proposition is based on the theory of Sokolov (1963) that the typical orienting response to a nonnoxious stimulus is digital vasoconstriction and cephalic vasodilation, while an intense or noxious stimulus produces a defensive response characterized by both digital and cephalic vasoconstriction. Feuerstein et al. (1982) have challenged these hypotheses by demonstrating vasodilation in response to stress in headache sufferers (migraine and tension) and controls and by citing other evidence that cephalic vasomotor reactivity to aversive stimulation is variable rather than consistently vasoconstriction. As a result of these observations, Feuerstein et al. (1982) argued that an earlier four-stage model of migraine may more adequately explain the relationship between stress and migraines. Tunis and Wolff (1953) observed that the temporal artery proceeded through a series of changes 36 to 72 hours preceding headache onset, including a shift from a steady state to (1) vasodilation with no associated pain 36 to 72 hours prior to the attack, (2) heightened lability 12 to 36 hours preceding headache, (3) vasoconstriction 6 hours prior to headache, and (4) vasodilation with concomitant pain.

Related to these models are a number of issues, the first of which is whether migraine is a tonic or phasic disorder (Morley, 1985). The former perspective views the vasomotor activity of migraine as abnormal between attacks and suggests that attacks are in some way exaggerations of this abnormality. The latter position characterizes migraine as a disorder in which abnormalities of function are seen only at times of headache attacks, which include prodromal and resolution phases; migraine attacks are assumed to be an idiosyncratic response to particular events. A second issue is whether the disorder is limited to the intra- and extracranial vessels or a more generalized dysfunction of vasomotor regulation.

Consideration of these models and issues emphasizes that some aspects of migraines are very difficult to investigate with currently available psychophysiological techniques. For example, psychophysiologists have no methods available for measuring intracranial blood flow. This is indeed a limitation, as a number of researchers have presented data suggesting that while intravascular factors operate for virtually all migraineurs, extracranial factors are present in only a proportion of cases (Blau & Dexter, 1981; Drummond & Lance, 1983).

Given the complexities of the models and issues, and the limitations of the available measurement techniques for exploring them, it is perhaps not surprising that although more than 20 studies have investigated the psychophysiology of migraine, no clear picture has yet emerged. Cardiovascular measures used in these studies have included temporal blood flow, which provides a direct index of the postulated vascular mechanism, as well as digital blood flow, facial and hand temperature, heart rate, and systolic and diastolic blood pressure. Although each of these measures provides unique information about the functioning of the cardiovascular system and therefore could help interpretation of temporal blood flow data, the measures have usually been included only as indicators of general arousal. Psychophysiologists investigating mechanisms of migraine have often resorted to the familiar paradigm of comparing groups of subjects at rest, in response to various stressors and tasks, and during "recovery" after the stressors or tasks, and it is these studies that will be reviewed first. It should be noted, however, that the relationship between this paradigm and mechanisms of migraine is often less than clear. For example, if headache-free migraineurs are compared with controls in terms of resting levels of cardiovascular variables, what results would be predicted? If the migraine subjects are more than 72 hours away from a headache, then whether any abnormality is predicted depends on whether a tonic or a phasic model is adopted. If subjects are within 72 hours of a migraine attack, then either vasodilation, heightened lability, or vasoconstriction might be predicted depending on which phase subjects are in at the time of measurement.

Considering first studies that have compared migraineurs with controls at rest, Morley (1985) reported significant elevations in variability of temporal blood flow and Philips and Hunter (1982a) found more abnormalities of temporal blood flow in migraineurs. Ahles et al. (1988) reported that migraineurs showed greater vasoconstriction of the left but not the right temporal artery than did controls. With respect to other cardiovascular variables, Drummond (1982) found elevated heart rate, diastolic blood pressure, and lower facial temperature on the side contralateral to the usual side of headache in migraineurs relative to controls. Significantly elevated heart rate was also reported by Passchier, van der Helm-Hylkema, and Orlebeke (1984a), with heart rate trends reported by Gannon, Haynes, Saffranek, and Hamilton (1981), Cohen, Williamson, et al. (1983), and Anderson and Franks (1981). The latter two studies also found trends for lower skin temperature in migraineurs. In contrast to these positive findings, other studies have found no significant differences between migraineurs and controls in terms of resting levels of cardiovascular variables (e.g., Feuerstein et al., 1982; Andrasik, Blanchard, Arena, Saunders, & Barron, 1982; Arena, Blanchard, Andrasik, Appelbaum, & Myers, 1985).

Studies comparing migraineurs with controls in response to stress seem to come closer to testing theories of migraine because they are relevant to the issue whether migraine is associated with exaggerated cranial artery responsiveness. Although results are not consistent, the literature includes a number of positive findings. Temporal vasodilation in migraineurs relative to controls has been demonstrated in response to noise (Rojahn & Gerhards, 1986), drinking ice water (McCaffrey, Goetsch, Robinson, & Isaac, 1986), and mental arithmetic (Drummond, 1982). Bakal and Kaganov (1977) reported decreased temporal pulse velocity in response to noise in migraineurs relative to controls and interpreted their data as indicating a vasoconstriction reaction in the headache group, but as discussed previously, a decrease in pulse velocity seems to suggest vasodilation not vasoconstriction. Morley (1985) demonstrated vasoconstriction in response to threat of noise in migraineurs compared to controls but pointed out that there was tentative evidence in his data for a tendency toward greater dilation at the pain site during the final seconds of the threat task (i.e., a rebound dilation). He suggested that the reason for the discrepancy between his finding of vasoconstriction and the finding of vasodilation by other researchers may be due to differences in the timing of measurement. His reported vasoconstriction took place in the first few seconds, while other researchers have reported stress responses over more prolonged periods. Other studies have failed to differentiate between migraineurs and controls in terms of vascular response to stress (e.g., Andrasik, Blanchard, Arena, Saunders, & Barron, 1982; Passchier et al., 1984a; Feuerstein et al., 1982).

In one of the few studies to compare migraineurs and controls in terms of poststress recovery, Gannon et al. (1981) reported significantly more vasoconstriction measured from the earlobe in the migraine group. Kroner-Herwig, Diergarten, Diergarten, and Seeger-Siewert (1988) found no differences between migraineurs and controls on four cardiovascular variables measured during poststress recovery, but they reported that migraineurs showed less digital vasodilation than did controls during a relaxation condition. A rather similar result was reported by Morley (1985), who found that migraineurs showed greater digital vasoconstriction and slower habituation rates during a "nonstressful" task (reaction-time task).

Our psychophysiological study involving pain induction and reduction procedures described in the section on tension headaches also included migraineurs (Martin, Marie, & Nathan, 1992). Results for the migraine group were similar to the tension headache group; in other words, migraineurs had distended superficial temporal arteries between pressure pulses, but not during the passage of pressure pulses, and had elevated blood pressure.

A variation on the stress reactivity studies is to test whether migraineurs evidence response stereotypy (Lacey, Kagen, Lacey, & Moss, 1962) consistent with vascular mechanisms. Response stereotypy refers to the hypothesized tendency of an individual to respond maximally and consistently in one particular physiological system. Cohen, Rickles, and McArthur (1978) demonstrated that migraineurs responded to a variety of stimulus situations with a more stereotyped, rigid response pattern across physiological systems than did control subjects. Additional support for response stereotypy in migraineurs has been demonstrated by Anderson, Stoyva, and Vaughn (1982), who showed that migraineurs consistently responded to different stressors in terms of elevated heart rate. Gannon et al. (1981) reported that migraineurs consistently responded across poststress recovery periods in terms of vasoconstriction measured from the earlobe. On the other hand, Kroner-Herwig et al. (1988) were unable to corroborate a specific vasomotor stress response stereotype in migraineurs.

One of the issues raised earlier in this section was whether migraine is a disorder of the intra- and extracranial arteries or a general dysfunction of vasomotor control. A number of studies have tried to answer this question but have produced conflicting findings. An early study by Appenzeller, Davison, and Marshall (1963) found an absence of normal reflex vasodilation in the hands of migraine patients in response to heating of the chest and concluded that this was evidence for a general peripheral vascular disorder among migraine sufferers. These results have been replicated by Downey and Frewin (1972) and Elliott, Frewin, and Downey (1973), but other researchers have found the peripheral reflex response of migraine sufferers and individuals not subject to migraines quite similar (French, Lassers, & Desai, 1967; Hockaday, Macmillan, & Whitty, 1967). In reviewing this literature, Morley (1977) concluded that the published studies have major methodological problems and there is no conclusive evidence that individuals subject to migraine have generalized vasomotor dysfunction.

One issue that has received little attention concerns the pain threshold of migraine sufferers. This is surprising considering that some theorists have invoked low threshold as a contributing factor. Wolff, Tunis, and Goodell (1953), for example, suggested that the pain of migraine was due to a combination of scalp tenderness and extracranial vasodilation. Three of the studies discussed earlier in the tension headache section also included migraineurs and their results did not differentiate the two headache types. Hence, Feuerstein et al. (1982) found no differences in pain threshold or tolerance (pressure stimuli applied to fingers) between migraineurs and controls, but Drummond (1987) demonstrated that migraineurs had significantly low thresholds (pressure stimuli applied to head) during headache and within

5 days of a headache but not at other times, and Schoenen et al. (1991) reported lower pressure–pain thresholds in migraineurs.

Another area that has not been explored extensively is comparisons between headache and headache-free states. This is unfortunate because such comparisons are central to the hypothesized vascular mechanism of migraine (i.e., head pain is postulated to be associated with vasodilation). The reason more attention has not been devoted to this type of analysis is probably the conviction held by many researchers referred to earlier, that such analyses are not valid with current psychophysiological techniques for measuring vasomotor activity. One exception is the study by Passchier et al. (1984a) which reported that migraineurs experiencing a headache had a significantly elevated heart rate relative to headache-free migraineurs. This study found no significant differences between these groups on a measure of temporal vasomotor activity but noted that the severity of pain states was mainly in the low range, as subjects were allowed to postpone experimental sessions if the pain was incapacitating.

Arena, Blanchard, Andrasik, Appelbaum, and Myers (1985) failed to differentiate migraineurs in headache versus headache-free conditions on any of the four psychophysiological variables analyzed but did not include their cephalic vasomotor data in this analysis because of concerns about its limitations. Similarly, Lichstein et al. (1991) compared migraineurs and controls during headache-free and headache sessions, in terms of forehead EMG, temporal BVP, and temporal and finger skin temperature, and failed to find any significant differences. A somewhat different approach was taken by Drummond and Lance (1983) who compared pulse amplitude data from the right and left temporal artery during unilateral migraine headaches. Analysis of the records of all subjects revealed no significant differences, but significant differences emerged from analysis of subgroups. Subjects whose headaches were confined to the frontotemporal area evidenced vasodilation on the headache side, as did subjects whose headaches were diminished via compression of the ipsilateral carotid artery.

In a study discussed earlier, I compared headache sufferers experiencing no headache, mild headache, and moderate headache across experimental conditions (Martin, Marie, & Nathan, 1992). We found a significant interaction between the state of dilation of the temporal artery between pressure pulses and experimental conditions. This interaction indicated that subjects with no headaches started the session with less dilated arteries than did subjects experiencing moderate headaches, but the gap between the groups narrowed as the experiment proceeded. Subjects with mild headaches showed an intermediate pattern of data.

A study by Friar and Beatty (1976) provided some tentative support for extracranial vasodilation as a pain mechanism of migraine by demonstrating that training to constrict the temporal artery resulted in a reduction in migraine attacks, while training subjects to constrict an artery at an irrelevant site (the hand) had no such effect. Similar findings were reported by Elmore and Tursky (1981) using hand temperature feedback as the control procedure. A subsequent study by Gauthier, Doyon, Lacroix, and Drolet (1983), however, questioned the interpretation of these findings. This study showed that training migraineurs to dilate the temporal artery was as effective for reducing headaches as training them to constrict the temporal artery, and both were significantly more effective than a waiting-list condition. Findings with respect to the relationship between BVP self-regulation skills and headache reduction are inconsistent, with reports of both significant findings (e.g., Lisspers & Ost, 1990a) and nonsignificant findings (e.g., Gauthier, Lacroix, Cote, Doyon, & Drolet, 1985).

Other Psychophysiological Mechanisms

Whereas the main focus of psychophysiological research investigating migraine mechanisms has been on cardiovascular variables, EMG (forehead, neck, temporalis, trapezius, and forearm), skin resistance, and respiration rate have also been measured in various studies. Studies comparing migraineurs and control subjects in terms of muscle tension have reported higher forehead EMG (e.g., Cohen, Williamson, et al., 1983; Philips, 1977b), neck EMG (e.g., Bakal & Kaganov, 1977; Pozniak-Patewicz, 1976), temporalis EMG (e.g., Philips, 1977b; Pozniak-Patewicz, 1976), and trapezius EMG (Ahles et al., 1988). On the other hand, many other studies have failed to find significant differences in EMG levels or EMG reactivity to stress between these two groups (e.g., Gannon et al., 1981; Anderson et al., 1982; Feuerstein et al., 1982; Andrasik, Blanchard, Arena, Saunders, & Barron, 1982; Rojahn & Gerhards, 1986; Passchier et al., 1984a).

Several studies have compared EMG levels between migraineurs and tension headache sufferers and Bakal and Kaganov (1977) reported higher levels in the former group. However, most studies have found no significant differences in EMG between the two headache types (e.g., Cohen, Williamson, 1983; Ahles et al., 1988; Martin, Marie, & Nathan, 1992).

Investigation of other variables has generally not led to significant findings. Two exceptions are the finding of Kroner-Herwig et al. (1988) that recovery from stress was delayed in migraineurs relative to controls in terms of skin resistance, and the finding of Drummond (1982) that migraineurs showed an elevated respiration rate compared to controls during isometric exercise.

Summary

Considering first the hypothesized muscular mechanism of tension headaches, the evidence is mixed but, on balance, quite unconvincing.

There is little support for the hypothesis that tension headache sufferers have generally elevated EMG levels or are slow to recover following stress. Higher muscle tension during headaches has not received consistent support. The evidence for headache sufferers responding to stress with more muscle tension than nonheadache sufferers is more promising, but many negative findings have been reported. It can be argued that the negative findings may result from investigators not using stressors that are personally relevant to the subjects or sufficiently aversive, but it can also be pointed out that a relatively subtle stress mechanism needs to be postulated to accommodate the common finding of normal levels of muscle tension during headaches. For example, the abnormal EMG response to stress would have to be conceptualized as a trigger for some other processes that cause or maintain head pain because tension levels do not appear to remain high during headaches.

One of the reasons it is hard to lend credence to muscular mechanisms of tension headaches is that it is difficult to explain away the large number of negative findings. In addressing this issue, Flor and Turk (1989) discuss procedural problems and variations in recording EMG that may account for the inconsistencies, but, as noted previously, EMG is relatively simple to monitor and the hypotheses linking muscle tension and headaches are straightforward to test. The positive findings that have been reported may have other interpretations than supporting a muscular mechanism for tension headaches. For example, they may arise as an artifact of inadequate matching of headache sufferers and controls, since the latter subjects have often been recruited from the investigator's colleagues or students who are more likely to be at ease (i.e., less tense) in a laboratory environment.

Of course, it is not possible to prove a null hypothesis so it cannot be stated categorically that tension headaches are not caused by contracted skeletal muscles. Perhaps the negative findings reflect recording from the wrong muscle sites or subjects in the wrong position. With respect to these possibilities, Hudzinski and Lawrence (1988) reported that tension headache sufferers did not display elevated EMG recorded from the commonly used forehead site but did display elevated EMG using the Schwartz–Mayo model (this placement purports to assess activity from the occipital area but seems likely to record activity from a wider area because it involves one active electrode on one frontalis muscle and the other active electrode on the ipsilateral posterior neck site, with the ground electrode on the side of the neck). Ahles et al. (1988) demonstrated that tension headache sufferers had normal trapezius EMG levels when measured in a reclining position but abnormalities in the sitting and standing positions. On the other hand, Hatch, Prihoda, Moore, and Cyr-Provost (1991) compared tension headache sufferers and nonheadache controls in terms of forehead and neck EMG recorded over periods of 48 to 96 hours in the natural environment. These authors found no difference in EMG levels between headache and control subjects and no evidence of elevated EMG during headache attacks.

Another approach to the negative findings is to argue that muscle tension causes headaches for some but not all tension headache cases, a position adopted by the IHS classification system. Haber, Kuczmierczyk, and Adams (1985), for example, split tension headache sufferers into high- and low-EMG groups following a screening session carried out while sufferers were experiencing headaches. The authors were able to show that the forehead EMG levels of the high-EMG group did differ from a control group and that systematic changes in EMG levels from headache to headache-free conditions occurred for the high-EMG group. Although the results of this study warrant further investigation, there is obviously a danger of circularity in selecting out a high-EMG subgroup and then demonstrating that it differs from an unselected control group. Ahles and Martin (1989) investigated the hypothesis that headache suffers with "normal" personality profiles as measured by the Minnesota Multiphasic Personality Inventory (MMPI) would evidence EMG and vasomotor abnormalities (i.e., have headaches that are primarily physiologically based) while patients with a "psychological disturbance" profile would demonstrate relatively less psychophysiological activity (i.e., headaches are more strongly related to psychological factors). Their results did not support such a dichotomy as more psychologically distressed subjects demonstrated higher forehead EMG.

Investigations of the vascular mechanism of migraine have also produced inconsistent findings but seem more promising. Comparisons of migraineurs and control subjects at rest suggest some temporal blood flow abnormalities such as increased variability and perhaps elevated cardiovascular arousal as indexed by heart rate and possibly other variables such as diastolic blood pressure and facial skin temperature. It is in the area of response to stress that the most impressive findings have occurred, however. Migraineurs evidence response stereotypy by responding maximally in terms of the cardiovascular system to a variety of stressors or conditions. In addition, relative to controls, migraineurs respond to stress with vasodilation of the temporal artery, possibly preceded by vasoconstriction. There is also some tentative evidence that migraineurs are slower to recover from stress. Distension of the arteries may occur between the passage of pressure pulses rather than during the passage of the pressure pulses. Whether migraine is a localized or a more generalized disorder of vasomotor regulation remains an open question.

In contrast to studies investigating muscular mechanisms of tension headaches, negative findings in this literature seem more likely to have occurred as a result of the formidable measurement problems discussed in this chapter. Other problems in this literature include uncertainties with respect to what is an "abnormal" response of the temporal artery to stress given that it is not clear what constitutes a "normal" response. Also, there are several variations of the vascular model and the main point of convergence of these models (intra- and extracranial dilation during headaches) is the one that presents the greatest measurement difficulties.

If muscle tension is not the critical causal factor of tension headaches, what is? A number of studies reviewed suggest that there are vascular abnormalities associated with tension headaches. Other studies have failed to differentiate psychophysiologically between tension headaches and migraines. If the mechanism of migraine is vascular this evidence also supports a vascular model of tension headaches. Parenthetically, if muscle tension is retained as a possible cause of tension headaches, the evidence suggests that muscle tension should also be considered a possible mechanism of migraine.

In summary, the psychophysiological findings pertaining to headache mechanisms are mixed. Currently, the evidence provides tentative support for all headaches being associated with vascular abnormalities. These abnormalities include variability of temporal artery blood flow and elevated cardiovascular arousal at rest, consistently responding to stress maximally with the cardiovascular system, and responding to stress with relatively distended temporal arteries. Pain thresholds for certain types of nociceptive stimuli in the region of the head may also be low for headache sufferers. A major problem in interpreting the psychophysiological data is determining whether abnormalities are a cause or an effect of headaches. Many of the abnormalities reviewed in this section, however, have occurred when the individuals were headache free, so the abnormalities could only be caused by headaches if being a chronic headache sufferer leads to abnormalities between headaches.

4

Antecedents and Consequences of Headaches

Antecedents

Immediate Factors

Some of the most obvious questions about immediate antecedents are: What proportion of headache sufferers can identify trigger factors, and how many trigger factors are typically identified? The answers to these questions are controversial. In his psychobiological model of chronic headaches, Bakal (1982) postulates that "the conditions controlling headache attacks in the chronic patient operate in a relatively autonomous fashion from both psychological and physical events that exist in the patient's environment" (p. 92). On the other hand, epidemiological studies indicate that approximately 85% of headache sufferers report at least one significant identifiable "cause" (Paulin et al., 1985; van den Bergh, Amery, & Waelkeins, 1987). Van den Bergh et al. (1987) found that migraineurs reported a median of three triggers with a range from 1 to 12; Blau and Thavapalan (1988) reported an average of four triggers volunteered by migraineurs, a number that increased to 5.5 with direct questioning.

Unfortunately, such data emerge from simplifying the complexities of headaches. Common responses of headache sufferers to whether factor X precipitates headaches are not yes or no but sometimes or possibly. Also, headache sufferes often decide that factor X does cause headaches and so they avoid factor X. This avoidance creates difficulties with respect to whether factor X does precipitate headaches. Some stimuli are reported as factors that do not trigger headaches but aggravate existent headaches, yet most studies do not take this distinction into account.

If one accepts that a number of factors can precipitate or aggravate headaches, questions are raised as to whether factors covary and interact with each other? Few studies have addressed these issues.

Papers relevant to immediate antecedents can be divided into four broad types on methodological grounds: clinical reports, retrospective studies, prospective studies, and manipulation studies. The literature review will be organized on the basis of these four categories, and studies considering factors individually will be discussed first, followed by those concerned with the relationship between factors.

CLINICAL REPORTS

Blau and Thavapalan (1988) note that an often expressed view is that "everything can produce a migraine" (p. 483). Precipitants listed in this study and by two other prominent clinicians in review articles (Diamond, 1979; Saper, 1978) include stress and emotional factors, poststress relaxation, exercise, fatigue, and too much or too little sleep. Foods considered triggers of migraine include ripened cheeses; herring; chocolate; vinegar; anything fermented, pickled, or marinated; sour cream and yogurt; nuts and peanut butter; hot fresh breads, raised coffe cakes, and doughnuts; pods of broad beans; any foods containing large amounts of monosodium glutamate; onions; canned figs; citrus foods; bananas; pizza; pork; excessive tea, coffee, and cola beverages; avocado; fermented sausage; chicken livers; and all alcoholic beverages. It has been suggested that withdrawal of reactive foods, particularly caffeine, may worsen headaches in the short term. It has also been suggested that headaches can be triggered by lack of food and smoking. Askmark, Lungberg, and Olsson (1989) reported a survey of drug-related headaches in which indomethacin (a nonsteroidal analgesic and anti-inflammatory agent used in the treatment of disorders such as rheumatoid arthritis and osteoarthritis) and nifedipine (a calcium antagonist used in the treatment and prevention of angina pectoris) were the drugs most frequently linked with headaches.

Menstrual factors can be important for female sufferers (headaches may be linked to before, during, or after periods). Perceptual factors that can act as triggers include visual stimuli such as glare, flicker, and eyestrain; noise; and smells. Seasonal and meteorological precipitants include cold, heat, humidity, and changes in weather. Other factors include allergies, neck pain, and sexual intercourse (benign orgasmic cephalalgia). Diamond (1979) draws attention to certain workers who are likely to suffer chronic headaches due to exposure to potentially toxic substances (e.g., auto mechanics who inhale carbon monoxide in a poorly ventilated garage).

A number of suggestions have been made as to how these precipitating factors may interact with each other. The occurrence of some factors may increase the likelihood of others occurring. For example, monthly hormonal changes in women may increase the probability of the consumption of certain foods (O'Banion, 1981). A number of authors have suggested that alcohol and food are more likely to trigger migraines at some times than at others (e.g., Saper, 1978; Dalton, 1975). Blau and Thavapalan (1988), for example, note that some women know that they can drink wine without inducing an attack except during the premenstrual week, and O'Banion (1981) argued that diet may influence the severity of problems produced by monthly menstrual cycles. Others have suggested that simultaneous exposure to more than one factor results in a multiplicative effect rather than an additive one (Leviton, 1984). Sauber (1980), for example, described the potentiating effect alcohol had on his headache vulnerability following consumption of monosodium glutamate ("Chinese restaurant" syndrome).

RETROSPECTIVE STUDIES

Retrospective studies have reported rates for trigger factors that vary considerably. Stress is the most commonly listed precipitant, with reported rates ranging from 17% (Paulin et al., 1985) to 61% (Drummond, 1985). Rates for menstruation vary from 6% (Phanthumchinda & Sithi-Amorn, 1989) to 48% (van den Bergh et al., 1987) for female headache sufferers. Some studies have reported rates of only a few percentage points for food as a trigger, but one early study reported that 25% of migraine sufferers experienced headaches precipitated by dietary factors such as fats, fried foods, chocolate, and oranges (Selby & Lance, 1960). One recent study reported rates of 27.5% for chocolate, 18.5% for cheese/dairy products, and 17% for fatty foods (van den Bergh et al., 1987). Reports of alcohol as a precipitant of headaches have varied from 0.6% (Paulin et al., 1985) to 51.6% (van den Bergh et al., 1987). High rates (i.e., above 10%) have been reported for fatigue (Paulin et al., 1985; van den Bergh et al., 1987), eyestrain (Vincent, Spierings, & Messinger, 1989; Paulin et al., 1985), glare (Drummond, 1985), heat (Levy, 1983), and seasonal and meteorological factors (Marrelli, Marini, & Prencipe, 1988; Zhao et al., 1988); lower rates (1% to 10%) have been reported, for noise and smoking (Paulin et al., 1985), hunger (Al-Rajeh, Bademosi, Ismail, & Awada, 1990), and exercise (Levy, 1983).

The differential prevalence rates probably reflect a multitude of factors, including genuine differences between countries and methodological differences between studies. With respect to the latter possibility, studies have inquired about antecedents in varied ways, including asking subjects to list precipitants and providing either short or long checklists. Stress seems an important factor across countries, but other factors appear more culturally bound. For example, alcohol was not listed as a precipitant of headaches in

Saudi Arabia (Al-Rajeh et al., 1990), witchcraft seemed a uniquely African precipitant (Levy, 1983), and sauna a rather Scandinavian phenomenon (Nikiforow & Hokkanen, 1978).

Given this diversity of reported headache triggers, we collected and factor-analyzed antecedent data to see whether meaningful patterns would emerge (Martin, Milech, & Nathan, 1992). Five factors were found, with Negative Affect accounting for the most variance. Stress (the most commonly reported precipitant), anxiety, depression, and anger correlated with the negative affect factor. Other factors were Visual Disturbance (flicker, glare, and eyestrain), Somatic Disturbance (sneezing, coughing, and pollen), Environmental Stress (humidity, high temperature, and opposite to relaxation), and Consumatory Stimuli (alcohol, food, and hunger). Tension headache versus migraine sufferers did not significantly differ in terms of negative affect or environmental stress, but migraineurs scored higher on visual disturbance, somatic stress, and consumatory stimuli. In other words, negative affect and environmental stress were equally common precipitants of both types of headaches, but the other antecedents were more likely to be endorsed by migraineurs.

PROSPECTIVE STUDIES

In an early prospective study of migraine precipitants, Henryk-Gutt and Rees (1973) asked 100 migraineurs to keep records of their migraine attacks and their emotional state at the time of the attack over 2 consecutive months. They found that 54% of migraine attacks coincided with emotional stress. Four more recent studies have analyzed the relationship between stress and headache. Sorbi and Tellegen (1988) reported a significant correlation ($r = .25$, $p < .001$) between threat as a form of everyday stress and occurrence of migraine attacks. Based on the Tunis and Wolff (1953) model discussed in Chapter 3 in which the buildup to a migraine takes place over 3 days, Levor, Cohen, Naliboff, McArthur, and Heuser (1986) compared the occurrence of stressful events over the 4 days leading up to and including a migraine day with the occurrence of stressful events over 4 headache-free days. Their data demonstrated significant elevations of stressful events and significant declines in physical activity in the 4 days associated with migraine. Kohler and Haimerl (1990) reported no increased stress for days 2 and 3 before a migraine attack but increased stress for the days immediately preceding and the days of an attack.

Mosley et al. (1990) investigated the relationship between stress and headaches using time-series analysis. They also based their methodology on the Tunis and Wolff (1953) model of migraine and calculated lagged correlations between headache activity and minor stressful life events recorded on 4 days (headache day and the preceding 3 days). Results indicated large in-dividual differences in the magnitude of stress–headache association (range of correlations from – .14 to .77). However, for a significant number of headache patients (60–70% tension headache and 39–46% migraine), stress accounted for 10% to 60% of the variance in headache activity over time. With respect to the temporal relationship between stress and headaches, headache activity was best predicted by stress occurring concurrently with headache for tension headache sufferers. For migraineurs, headache activity was best predicted by stress that occurred 1 to 3 days earlier.

Other studies have investigated the relationship between headaches and mood. Harvey and Hay (1984) reported that migraineurs were significantly more depressed on headache days than on days preceding the headache. Other negative moods such as tension, discontent, and lethargy also seemed heightened in subjects on headache days. Harrigan, Kues, Ricks, and Smith (1984) calculated correlations between headaches and 10 mood states mea-sured at the time of headache for periods ranging from 12 to 36 hours prior to headache in migraineurs. In general, correlations between same-period mood and headaches showed a stronger relationship than those for lagged mood ratings. Feelings of constraint and fatigue produced the highest corre-lations with headaches ranging from .31 to .36 when recorded during the evening or night of a headache. In a similar vein, Arena, Blanchard, and Andrasik (1984) calculated correlations between headaches and three moods (anxiety, hunger, and depression) measured during five periods (headache day, 1 day before, 2 days before, 1 day after, and 2 days after). Again, the highest correlations were with same-day mood, but the correlations were all low (correlation averaged across the three moods of $r = .16$, $p < .09$).

In one of my studies (Martin, Nathan, Milech, & van Keppel, 1988), we found headaches to be significantly associated with all six moods measured (anxiety, hostility, depression, unsureness, tiredness, and confusion), with little difference in strength of associations. As with the other studies, correla-tions between mood and headaches were higher for same-day mood than for day-before mood or day-after mood. Individual differences in the association between headaches and mood were very large, however, paralleling the finding of Mosley et al. (1990) for headaches and stress. Multiple regression analyses were performed for each subject to determine how well headache status could be predicted from all six mood states. Correlations varied dramat-ically from a subject whose six correlations ranged from −.85 to −.98 (mood accounting for 97% of the variance in headache versus headache free) to a subject whose correlations ranged from .11 to .35 (mood accounting for 18% of the variance). Also, individuals varied in terms of which mood was most closely associated with their headaches.

The only other antecedent factor to be studied via a prospective design is food intake. Dalton (1975) asked migraineurs to complete forms each time a migraine attack occurred over a 3-month period. The forms required details of all food and drink consumed during the 24 hours immediately prior to the attack. She reported that a dietary factor was isolated in 95% of 2,313 attacks studied. Consumption of cheese occurred prior to 40% of attacks, with the corresponding figures for chocolate, alcohol, and citrus foods being 33%, 23%, and 21%, respectively. Fasting (5 hours a day or 13 hours overnight) occurred prior to 67% of attacks.

Medina and Diamond (1978) requested migraineurs to self-monitor diet and headaches and found that some headaches were time-locked to the intake of alcoholic drinks, chocolate, and fasting but less so to citrus and nuts.

MANIPULATION STUDIES

Many studies have manipulated stress in headache sufferers and hence can be argued to be relevant to the relationship between stress and headaches. All these studies, however, with two exceptions, have focused on the effect of stress on physiological variables rather than on headache activity. If the physiological response to stress of headache sufferers differs from the response of controls, this difference constitutes indirect evidence in support of a relationship between stress and headaches. As reviewed in Chapter 3, the data with respect to stress responses are inconsistent.

The only two studies that have directly investigated the effect of stress on headaches were mentioned in the previous chapter. Gannon et al. (1987) exposed headache and control subjects to a 1-hour cognitive stressor (mental arithmetic with failure feedback) and reported that six of eight tension headache subjects, five of eight migraineurs, and two of eight control subjects developed headaches during the stress period. Using the same stressor, Haynes et al. (1990) found that 30 out of 36 subjects in a mixed headache sample reported a headache during the procedure.

In one of my studies on mood and headaches (Martin et al., 1988), we used the musical mood-induction procedure to induce despondency and happiness in headache and control subjects. This manipulation provided some support for mood as a causal influence on headaches because the happiness condition was associated with a significant decrease in headache intensity and the despondency condition tended to be associated with an increase in headache intensity. These findings seem noteworthy since the mood-induction procedure used was only 7 minutes in duration.

Some headache treatments have been specifically designed to help suf-ferers cope with stress, while many others seem likely to have this effect (e.g., relaxation training). Stress-reduction approaches to headaches have had some success. The success of such treatments provides some weak, indirect support for a stress–headache relationship. The results of such studies are reviewed in the next chapter.

The headache precipitant that has received the most attention after stress and mood is food. The dietary factor most commonly reported by patients as a precipitant of headaches is chocolate (Blau & Diamond, 1985). Moffett, Swash, and Scott (1974) investigated the effect of chocolate in migraine by carrying out two separate double-blind studies on migraineurs who had observed that headaches regularly occurred after the ingestion of small amounts of cocoa products. The two studies involved a total of 80 dietary challenges and headaches were reported following eating chocolate on 13 occasions, eating placebo on 8 occasions, and eating both on 2 occasions. The results suggest that chocolate on its own is rarely a precipitant of migraine. Koehler and Glaros (1988) completed a double-blind randomized crossover study comparing the effect of aspartame (dietary sweetener) to that of matched placebo on migraine headache. The results indicated that the ingestion of aspartame caused a significant increase in headache frequency for some subjects.

Medina and Diamond (1978) randomly assigned 24 migraineurs, 18 of whom thought that one or more foodstuffs were related to their headaches, to three diets. Diet A involved consuming considerable amounts of food with high content in tyramine and other vasoactive substances (phenylethylamine, nitrate, and levodopa) every day and avoiding other foodstuffs known to contain none or insignificant amounts of these substances. Diet B involved the reverse of Diet A, and Diet C consisted of eating and drinking ad lib. All subjects rotated through the three diets following each for a period of 6 weeks while monitoring headaches and diet. The results showed no significant differences in indices of migraine or headache medication between the three diets.

Studies treating headaches by using elimination diets have produced impressive results. O'Banion (1981) reported five case studies of individuals experiencing migraine, tension headache, or combined headaches treated by controlling dietary factors using an A-B-A-C single-case experimental design. Headaches were eliminated in four of five cases. Grant (1979) reported on 60 migraineurs who completed elimination diets after a 5-day period of withdrawal from their normal diet. When an average of 10 common foods were avoided, there was a dramatic fall in the number of headaches per month; 85% patients became headache free. Scopp (1991) treated two individuals, both suffering from migraine and tension headache, by eliminating all food sources containing monosodium glutamate. Marked reductions in the frequency of both types of headaches were reported for both cases. Radnitz, Blanchard, and Bylina (1990) treated two migraineurs who had failed to respond to stress management training via a dietary approach. After elimination of trigger foods, both individuals showed a 50% decrease in headache activity.

Blau and Cumings (1966) investigated the effect of fasting on migraine by comparing headaches on 2 days: on 1 day fasting took place for 19 hours; on the other subjects ate and drank normally. No headaches developed on the control days, but 6 out of 12 subjects experienced a migraine attack on the fast day, and another 3 developed headaches, one of these occurring the next day.

Evidence pertaining to the relationship between visual factors and headaches is limited. Wilkins et al. (1984) reported that subjects who complained of frequent headaches were more likely to experience significant discomfort and visual distortion while viewing black-and-white-striped gratings than were subjects without headaches. Moreover, stripe viewing induced headache attacks in some subjects with a headache history. Similarly, Marcus and Soso (1989) found that 82% of migraineurs demonstrated stripe aversion whereas only 6.2% without migraine evidenced stripe discomfort. Also, in 3 out of 38 migraineurs, migraine symptoms were induced within several hours of stripe viewing. Drummond (1986) studied photophobia in migraineurs, tension headache sufferers, and controls. He reported that subjective estimates of glare and light-induced pain were greatest in patients with migraine at the time of examination, but ratings by tension headache sufferers also exceeded control ratings at most levels of illumination.

Other studies that involve manipulation of single hypothesized headache antecedents have reported effects only in terms of sensitivity and physiological reactions rather than establishing direct links with headache activity. Rojahn and Gerhards (1986), for example, demonstrated that migraineurs rated a loud shrill noise as more aversive than did control subjects. Also, the migraineurs and controls differed with respect to temporal BVP recorded during the noise stimulation. Similarly, Bakal and Kaganov (1977) found a decrease in blood flow velocity recorded from the temporal arteries in response to noise by both tension headache and migraine subjects but the opposite response in controls. McCaffrey et al. (1986) investigated response to consumption of ice water and reported markedly differential responding in terms of BVP between migraine and control subjects.

One study has investigated the effects of manipulating multiple antecedent factors on headaches. Lai, Dean, Ziegler, and Hassanein (1989) recruited a group of subjects with a history of diet-induced migraine and (1) instructed them to fast for 12 hours before attending their laboratory, (2) asked them to consume red wine, chocolate, and cheese in the laboratory, and (3) exposed them to photic stimulation and hyperventilation. Headaches occurred in 42% of the sample.

In contrast to Lai et al.'s use of multiple factors to induce headaches, Blau and Thavapalan (1988) treated migraineurs by encouraging them to avoid precipitating factors. This reduced attacks from two to one per month in 19 of the 23 subjects, and lessened severity or better analgesic control was noted by some subjects. Dalton (1973) has also reported successful treatment of migraine cases by eliminating trigger factors.

Setting Factors

STRESS

Review of the literature on factors that precipitate or aggravate headaches provides some support for stress as a trigger. From a practitioner's perspective, this finding leads clinicians to want to understand why their patients experience stress when they do, because understanding may suggest appropriate intervention strategies. From the related research perspective, the finding raises many issues concerning the etiology of stress-induced headaches, such as whether individuals who suffer from regular headaches differ from individuals who do not in terms of exposure to stressors or to the factors that mediate the stress response. More specifically, questions relating to headache sufferers versus nonheadache controls include: Do headache sufferers differ in terms of major life stresses or everyday stresses, appraisal of stressful events, coping strategies to manage stressful events, and perceived social support?

A number of studies have investigated stressful life events experienced by recurrent headache sufferers and controls during periods ranging from 1 month to 2 years and found no significant differences (Andrasik, Blanchard, Arena, Teders, Teevan et al., 1982; Andrasik & Holroyd, 1980b; Martin & Theunissen, 1992). Invernizzi, Gala, and Sacchetti (1985) found no difference between a headache and a control group in terms of incidence of stressful events in early life. However, the headache group had experienced a greater incidence of stressful events during the year before headache onset. Holm, Holroyd, Hursey, and Penzien (1986) reported a statistically significant difference between tension headache sufferers and controls in terms of life events in the previous month, but the difference only amounted to headache sufferers experiencing on average one more stressful event. Differences between the groups were much more apparent in terms of daily hassles. Headache sufferers reported seven more daily hassles in the previous month than did controls. De Bededittis and Lorenzetti (in press) also reported a relationship between daily hassles and headaches but not life events and headaches. Martin and Soon (1992) found significantly higher perceived stress in headache sufferers relative to nonheadache controls.

Holm et al. (1986) also found that headache sufferers appraised the stressful events they experienced more negatively than did controls. Specifically, when the potential impact of a stressful event was ambiguous, headache sufferers perceived the event as having greater impact and themselves as having less control over the event than did controls. In addition, headache sufferers employed less effective coping strategies in their efforts to manage stressful events since they placed more reliance on the relatively ineffective coping strategies of avoidance and self-blame and made less use of social support than did controls. A recent follow-up study confirmed that sufferers of both migraine and tension headache appraised and coped with stressful events differently from headache-free controls (Ehde & Holm, 1992).

In two studies comparing headache sufferers with matched nonheadache controls, we have found headaches to be associated with deficits in perceived social support. Martin and Theunissen (1992) reported differences between headache and control groups in terms of availability and adequacy of attachment and availability and adequacy of social integration. Martin and Soon (1992) found headache sufferers were significantly less satisfied with the support available to them and scored lower on all four types of functional support measured in the study: appraisal support, esteem support, belonging support, and tangible support.

Studies considered so far have examined the relationship between headaches and stress generally. A few papers have looked at the relationship between headaches and particular life circumstances that are likely to give rise to stress. Kunzer (1987), for example, investigated marital adjustment and headaches and found that headache sufferers and their spouses scored significantly lower on the Dyadic Adjustment Scale (DAS) than did the well-adjusted couples reported in the test norms. Twenty-five percent of the headache sample attained scores that indicated marital distress. Roy (1986) discussed the role of marital conflict in exacerbating headaches and described four illustrative cases. Family therapy was used to treat these cases with mixed results. Featherstone and Beitman (1984) claimed that daily migraine is a response to marital stress and outlined a four-stage process by which "marital migraine" develops.

EMOTIONAL STATES

If emotional factors such as anxiety and depression can precipitate or aggravate headaches, then negative emotional states can be viewed as risk factors for headaches. That is, individuals who experience negative affect, which in its extreme form constitutes emotional or mood disorders, are particularly vulnerable to headaches precipitated by affective factors.

Numerous authors have commented on the frequent coexistence of headaches and the symptoms of emotional disorders. Lance (1973) stated that in his experience, approximately one third of patients with tension headaches have symptoms of depression. In a study of 500 migrainous patients, Selby and Lance (1960) found overt symptoms of anxiety in 13% of their sample, one third of whom were subject to depression at times other than their migraine attacks. Kashiwagi, McLure, and Wetzel (1972) reported that investigation of 100 cases of functional headaches revealed that 50% were suffering from depressive syndrome. Dalessio (1972) has argued that "chronic headache may serve to obscure a serious emotional disorder, most often a depression. . . . Anxiety and especially depression symptoms are converted into acceptable (to the patient) physical symptoms" (pp. 548–549). Featherstone (1985) found that depression or anxiety was significantly more commonly diagnosed in headache sufferers than in matched controls; Morrison and Price (1989) reported that 33% of referrals to a migraine clinic met the *Diagnostic and Statistical Manual of Mental Disorders*, third edition (DSM-III) criteria for affective disorder.

A number of studies have administered depression, anxiety, and anger inventories to headache sufferers and controls. These studies overlap investigations of personality traits in headache sufferers, which are reviewed in a subsequent section. Philips and Hunter (1982b) administered the Wakefield Depression Scale to 300 randomly selected psychiatric patients and found significantly higher scores in those who suffered from headaches than those who did not. I administered the Beck Depression Inventory (BDI) to headache sufferers and controls and found significantly higher scores in the former group (Martin, Nathan, Milech, & van Keppel, 1988). Inspection of the categories into which the scores fell indicated that the majority of headache sufferers (56%) were not severely depressed; the group differences occurred in the mildly to moderately depressed categories, which accounted for 41% of the headache subjects compared to only 17% of the controls. Price and Blackwell (1980) administered the Taylor Manifest Anxiety Scale to migraineurs and controls and found significantly higher scores in the former group. Andrasik and Holroyd (1980b) reported that a tension headache sample scored higher on the Spielberger Trait Anxiety Inventory than a nonheadache control group. A recent study by Hatch, Schoenfeld et al., (1991) compared tension headache sufferers and controls and found the former to have higher levels of anxiety, depression, and anger/hostility.

OTHER FACTORS

It seems likely that many factors other than stress and emotions can act as setting factors for headaches. For example, if an individual's headaches were precipitated or aggravated by visual stimuli such as flicker, glare, and eyestrain, a work situation that necessitated spending much time looking at a video display terminal (VDT) screen might be construed as a setting factor for that individual's headaches. Setting factors may follow weekly, monthly, or yearly cycles. Exposure to immediate antecedents such as stress and diet are likely to vary between weekdays and weekends, for example, providing opportunities for cyclical variation in headaches. Menstrual factors have been discussed under the heading of immediate antecedents but may act as setting factors for some female headache sufferers. Meteorological and seasonal factors vary through the year, perhaps resulting in changing vulnerability to headaches.

Data relevant to these possibilities are generally not available. One exception is a study by Brewerton and George (1990) which reviewed admissions to a hospital in South Carolina for migraine over a 20-year period. These authors reported that admissions peaked in spring for female patients, an effect that was absent in male patients. A retrospective survey by Marelli et al. (1988) also suggested a high incidence of classic migraine associated with spring.

Onset Factors

It was noted in Chapter 2 that headaches can begin early in life but that 80–90% have onset between ages 10 and 40. It would seem likely that headache onset may be sudden or gradual and could be related to a variety of psychological or biological processes or events. Learning processes such as modeling and operant and classical conditioning appear potentially important, particularly in cases of headache onset during childhood. Very little data have been published, however, relating to onset factors.

The belief that stressful events may lead to onset of headaches is an old one. Wolff (1937), for example, found that events such as vacations, examinations, increased responsibility, criticism, and fear of failure have all been associated with headache onset. While acknowledging the difficulty of determining whether headache onset was related to stress, Howarth (1965) reported that stress factors seemed relevant in 54% of cases. The stress factors were divided into domestic and social problems (28%), occupational difficulties (19%), and fear of illness (7%). A similar relationship was reported by Henryk-Gutt and Rees (1973), who found that psychological stress was evident at onset of first migraine for 50% of their sample. Domino and Haber (1987) investigated physical and sexual abuse in women presenting to a pain center with chronic headaches. They found a high incidence of such abuse (66% of sample) and reported that head pain developed after trauma in 100% of these cases.

Weiss, Stern, and Goldberg (1991) reported on a series of 35 headache sufferers with no prior history of headaches who developed recurrent episodic headaches following a minor head or neck injury.

The only other onset factors that have received attention are specifically female ones that are believed to be hormonally mediated, namely, menarche, use of oral contraceptives, and pregnancy (Hering & Rose, 1992). Menarche is considered by some to be associated with the onset or exacerbation of headaches. Kudrow (1978) argued that the female-to-male ratio of migraine in children is 1:1 but that the female rate increases, thus changing the ratio to 2:1. Ziegler (1978) reviewed data indicating that the preponderance of migraine in females begins at age 11 and that migrainous women tend to show striking decreases in migraine with menopause. On the other hand, Deubner (1977) found that the menarchal status of his female sample ages 10 to 20 years was not related to the onset of migraine or other headache and suggested that the role of hormonal changes in the onset of headache was probably minimal.

Carroll (1971) reported that the use of oral contraceptives tends to increase the frequency of migraine headaches in women. Kudrow (1975) found a greater number of headaches reported in female migraineurs who were taking estrogen containing contraceptives or were on estrogen maintenance than in female migraineurs using no hormones. Kudrow also reported that in 70% of those cases in which birth control pills were discontinued, a reduction in the frequency of migraine headaches was observed; when a 50% reduction in estrogen intake was initiated in the estrogen maintenance group, 58% of cases reported a reduction in headache frequency.

A number of studies have reported that headaches commonly are relieved during pregnancy—particularly, but not exclusively, for women whose headaches had previously occurred during menses (e.g., Epstein, Hockaday, & Hockaday, 1975; Callaghan, 1968). These studies suggest a remission or improvement rate of 60–80% in migraine headaches during pregnancy. On the other hand, migraine sometimes occurs for the first time during pregnancy particularly in the first trimester (e.g., Chancellor, Wroe, & Cull, 1990; Uknis & Silberstein, 1991). This is relatively rare, however, occurring in 4–10% of cases, and the prognosis of such individuals is good so they are likely to present infrequently in chronic headache samples.

Predisposing Factors

FAMILIAL INCIDENCE

Migraine has long been accepted as a family condition, and in fact many neurologists consider a family history to be a prerequisite for the diagnosis of migraine (Ziegler, 1978). Early studies reported high concordance rates, with Allan (1930) finding a history of migraine in one or both parents in 91.4% of migraine patients and Goodell, Lewontin, and Wolff (1954) reporting that 84% of migrainous patients had at least one relative with migraine. However, more recent studies have found much lower rates of concordance. Ziegler (1978) reviewed three studies that reported positive family history for headaches in migraineurs versus controls as 61% (parents only) versus 11% (parents only); 36.5% versus 5.8%; and 72.6% (mothers) and 20.5% (fathers) versus 17.8% (parents or siblings).

Even more extreme is a study by Waters (1971) that reported a prevalence of migraine in the family of migraine patients of 10%, compared to 5% and 6% in the families of nonmigrainous headache and nonheadache groups, respectively. This difference was not statistically significant. Waters pointed out that other studies have contained possible biases, in particular, the one that accepted a case as migraine if there is a positive family history. Also, most studies have asked subjects to indicate the degree of familial incidence of headaches, but in the study by Waters first-degree relatives were contacted directly.

GENETICS OF HEADACHES

The early studies reporting high concordance rates for migraine led a number of authors to suggest that migraine was an inherited disorder. Goodell et al. (1954), for example, concluded their paper with the summary statement, "Highly significant evidence has been offered demonstrating the hereditary character of migraine and permitting one further to assume correctly that the inheritance of the migraine headache trait is through a recessive gene with a penetrance of approximately 70%" (p. 33). Other authors have argued that migraine is due to a dominant gene (Allan, 1930; Christiansen, 1925) or numerous genes (Dalsgaard-Nielsen, 1965). Not surprisingly, Waters (1971) drew a rather different conclusion after finding much lower concordance rates. He suggests that "family history should not be included in the definition of migraine and that heredity is much less important in migraine than is usually supposed" (p. 77). On the basis of a segregation analysis of migraine in families, Devoto et al. (1986) suggested the existence of a possible genetic heterogeneity of liability to migraine.

Of course, studies of family occurrence do not separate the contributions of heredity versus environment on pathology. Investigations of concordance rates in monozygotic (MZ) and dizygotic (DZ) twins come closer to this goal. In reviewing previous twin studies of migraine, Lucas (1977) tabulated concordance rates varying from 14% to 100% for MZ twins and from 0% to 40% for DZ twins. All but one of these studies used very small samples (i.e., less than 20 twin pairs), and it is noticeable that all four of the studies reporting 100% concordance were studies of only a few twins (i.e., 1 to 5 pairs). In Lucas's own, much larger study (161 twin pairs) he found a concordance rate of 26% for MZ twins and 13% for DZ twins, a difference that was statistically significant. Lucas concluded, like Waters, that his findings suggested a much lower genetic factor in migraine than previously thought.

Of course, even twin studies do not fully disentangle heredity versus environmental factors, because the environment of MZ twins is likely to be more similar than the environment of DZ twins. Hence, adoption studies are needed in which probrands and cosiblings who have been reared apart are assessed for concordance, but this type of study has not been carried out with headache sufferers.

Ziegler (1978) has pointed out that "whatever may be inherited is clearly not a headache, but rather a type of physiological or psychological reaction to various environmental influences" (p. 30). Unfortunately, precisely what is inherited is quite unclear, although Ziegler suggests possibilities that have arisen out of research findings such as vasomotor instability (Appenzeller et al., 1963) or reaction of the central nervous system to photic stimuli (Richey, Kooi, & Waggoner, 1966).

PERSONALITY

One approach to inherited predisposition is to consider whether individuals with particular personality traits or profiles are more vulnerable to headaches, since personality is partially genetically determined. Given the literature reviewed so far, it seems likely that at least some form of relationship between headaches and personality characteristics exists. If common precipitants of headaches are anxiety, anger, and depression, for example, individuals who experience these emotions regularly (i.e., are high on the corresponding personality traits) are likely to be predisposed to headaches.

For many years it has been argued that headache sufferers tend to have a particular personality profile (Harrison, 1975). Descriptions of the personality traits that characterize migraine have been remarkably consistent. Henryk-Gutt and Rees (1973), for example, suggested the prevalent view of a migraine sufferer as "a tense, driving, obsessional perfectionist with an inflexible personality, who maintains a store of bottled-up resentments which can neither be expressed nor resolved. These characteristics would make him (or more often her) unable to adapt easily to circumstances, but liable to react excessively to environmental and interpersonal stresses sometimes with a migraine attack" (p. 142). Fewer descriptions of the personality traits associated with tension headaches have appeared in the literature, but those that have share much in common with the migraine profile. Martin (1966), for example, described tension headache patients as "sensitive, perfectionistic, worrisome, chronically tense and apprehensive" (p. 49).

The literature on personality and headaches is extensive as exemplified by a review of this area by Blanchard, Andrasik, and Arena (1984). These authors tracked down 67 studies that they characterized as primarily observational and a further 38 investigations that employed standardized psychological tests, in addition to their own studies. Hence, this review will necessarily be selective, focusing on the more recent and better controlled studies with an emphasis on the major issues in the field.

A study lauded by Blanchard et al. (1984) as coming closest to being a model investigation in this field was carried out by Kudrow and Sutkus (1979). These authors compared six headache types on the MMPI and found three significantly distinct groups: Group A, migraine and cluster headache; Group B, tension and combined headache; and Group C, posttraumatic and conversion headache. They proposed a continuum of psychopathology with Group A as the most normal and Group C the most neurotic. They reported that 75% to 80% of patients could be assigned to these three groups, on the basis of their scores on scales 1 (Hypochondriasis, or somatic preoccupation), 2 (Depression), and 3 (Hysteria, or denial) of the MMPI. Other results from this study included the finding of a significant "conversion V" pattern (also known as the "neurotic triad" and comprising clinically significant elevations on scales 1, 2, and 3) in women with tension, posttraumatic, and conversion headaches and in men with combined headache. The often reported characteristics of perfectionism and rigidity were not present in this sample of migraineurs.

Sternbach, Dalessio, Kunzel, and Bowman (1980) supported the findings of Kudrow and Sutkus that migraineurs tended to be less neurotic than the other headache groups and those with tension headaches more so, but they found somewhat different patterns and interpreted the results differently. They suggested that MMPI differences between diagnostic groups may be related to "pain density." The higher scores exhibited in the profiles of tension and combined headache sufferers may be because these individuals experience fewer pain-free intervals than do migraineurs.

Andrasik, Blanchard, Arena, Teders, and Rodichok (1982) reported a cross-validation analysis of the Kudrow–Sutkus MMPI classification system with mixed results. A high level of support for Group A was obtained but a low level of support for Group B. Andrasik, Blanchard, Arena, Teders, and Rodichok (1982) pointed out that their data suggested that none of the headache groups was characterized by marked elevations in any of the extensive battery of psychological tests used in their study.

A recent study by Dieter and Swerdlow (1988) of the Kudrow–Sutkus classification system resulted in only 40% correct classification. Conversion V patterns occurred in a significantly greater degree of headache patients than in controls, but the percentage of occurrence ranged from only 13% to 31%.

The studies considered so far have all employed the MMPI to assess personality, but many other standardized instruments have been used. Using a battery of five tests, Passchier, van der Helm-Hylkema, and Orlebeke

(1984b) showed that tension headache and migraine cases had elevated achievement motivation and tension headache cases demonstrated greater rigidity. They found no evidence of higher neuroticism, obsessive–compulsive behavior, or abnormal patterns of defense mechanisms. In contrast, Blaszczynski (1984) reported higher levels of neuroticism and repressed hostility in female migraine and tension headache sufferers not attending clinics than in no-pain controls, but equally elevated levels were present in a "pain" control group (chronic or recurring pain but no complaint of headache). No evidence for increased incidence of obsessionality was found.

Arena, Blanchard, Andrasik, and Applebaum (1986) compared three kinds of headache sufferer and noheadache controls in terms of obsessiveness and compulsivity. They found few differences between the groups, thus replicating the findings by Passchier et al. (1984b) and Blaszczynski (1984). In addition, the data from this study failed to support the construct of a pain density function in headaches, although previous work by the same authors did demonstrate support (Andrasik, Blanchard, Arena, Teders, Teevan, & Rodichok, 1982).

In reviewing this literature, Blanchard et al. (1984) concluded that the data do not support the notion of a "headache personality." They do suggest, however, that chronic headache sufferers as a group are more psychologically distressed and show more "deviant personality characteristics" than do nonheadache sufferers, and that on most measures it is the tension headache sufferers who are most discrepant. Similar conclusions were reached by Williams, Thompson, Haber, and Raczynski (1986).

Since publication of these reviews, researchers have continued to look for a migraine personality but with little success (e.g., Hundleby & Loucks, 1985; Schmidt, Carney, & Fitzsimmons, 1986). One interesting development, however, has been the application of the Type A personality or behavior pattern construct to headache sufferers. Since the Type A behavior pattern is similar to descriptions of the migraine personality, and since it is certainly a risk factor for coronary heart disease (e.g., Blumenthal, Williams, Kong, Schonberg, & Thompson, 1978; Haynes, Feinleib, & Kannel, 1980) and possibly a more general health risk factor (e.g., Review Panel, 1981; Woods & Burns, 1984), a number of researchers have explored the relationship between headaches and the Type A behavior pattern.

Hicks and Campbell (1983) administered the Jenkins Activity Schedule (JAS) to a student sample and found that Type A's experienced significantly more tension headaches and migraines than did Type B's. Similarly, Woods, Morgan, Day, Jefferson, and Harris (1984) reported that the increasing frequency of both migraine and tension headache was significantly associated with higher scores on the Type A scale of the JAS. Martin, Nathan, and Milech (1987), using the Framingham Type A questionnaire, demonstrated that students who suffered from more frequent headaches and headaches of higher intensity have significantly elevated Type A scores. They also showed that the majority of chronic headache sufferers displayed the Type A behavior pattern. Unfortunately, two more recent studies have suggested a much weaker link between headaches and the Type A behavior pattern (Hillhouse, Blanchard, Appelbaum, & Kirsch, 1988; Rappaport, McAnulty, & Brantley, 1988).

Another interesting recent development was the finding by Passchier, Schouten, van der Donk, and van Romunde (1991) of an interaction between personality characteristics and life events. Subjects in this study with at least weekly headaches had more life events and higher inadequacy, social inadequacy, rigidity, and injuredness than did subjects with less frequent headaches. Significant interactions were reported between life events and all four of these personality charracteristics for younger subjects (under 50). The interaction between inadequacy and life events was also significant for older subjects.

Even the conclusion reached by Blanchard et al. (1984) that chronic headache sufferers show more deviant personality characteristics has to be tempered in a number of ways. First, it is unclear whether the findings supporting this conclusion are an artifact of subject selection or measurement instruments. Philips (1976), for example, has pointed out that more than 50% of headache sufferers do not seek medical advice, and individuals who complain to their doctors have a particular type of personality characterized by extraversion and neuroticism (Bond & Pilowsky, 1966). Hence, clinicians see an unrepresentative sample of headache sufferers. This argument was supported by Philips' own data which showed that headache sufferers selected from a community sample without reference to headache complaints made to their doctors were not significantly different from the test norms on neuroticism, extraversion, or psychoticism. In contrast, female tension headache cases selected on the basis of the severity of their headaches and their desire for treatment showed significantly elevated neuroticism.

The importance of subject recruitment procedures was also emphasized in a study by McAnulty et al. (1986) in which they demonstrated that subjects who responded promptly to advertisements exhibited significantly higher levels of psychopathology than did later volunteers. Blanchard et al. (1984) noted that most of the available data had been collected at specialty clinics and therefore may be biased in the direction of exaggerated psychopathology.

With respect to measurement artifacts, Dieter and Swerdlow (1988) have pointed out that elevation on certain MMPI scales, particularly those that reflect somatic overconcern, may be the result of measuring headache symptomatology rather than psychopathology. In support of this suggestion, Dieter and Swerdlow rescored data from scales 1 and 3 of the MMPI in their study after removing headache-associated items. This resulted in statistically and clinically significant reductions in scores on these scales. The point that these authors make about the MMPI is equally valid for many of the other instruments used by researchers in this field.

Another factor that needs to be considered with respect to concluding that chronic headaches are associated with deviant personality characteristics is whether the characteristics are uniquely linked to headaches or associated with other health problems also. This concern is reinforced by the study discussed earlier in which headache sufferers differed from no-pain controls but not pain controls (Blaszczynski, 1984). Similarly, Blanchard, Radnitz et al. (1986) reported that tension headache sufferers and migraineurs were more psychologically distressed than normals but less distressed than an irritable-bowel syndrome group.

Friedman and Booth-Kewley (1987) carried out a meta-analytic review of the literature on personality correlates of five diseases with psychosomatic components: headaches, asthma, arthritis, ulcers, and coronary heart disease. Their results point to the probable existence of a generic disease-prone personality that involves depression, anger/hostility, anxiety, and possibly other aspects of personality. However, except in the case of coronary heart disease, the evidence was weak.

The final factor meriting consideration with respect to the association between chronic headaches and deviant personality characteristics is whether the relationship is causal, and if causal, in which direction. It is quite plausible that rather than personality traits or profiles predisposing individuals to headaches, deviant personality characteristics and headaches both result from an unidentified pathological process, or that the experience of living with pain causes personality changes. These possibilities are not mutually exclusive and psychopathology may function as both a cause and a consequence of headaches (Collet, Cottraux, & Juenet, 1986). The possibility of psychological distress as a consequence of headaches is consistent with studies by Sternbach and Timmermans (1975) and Merskey (1972) which presented evidence that chronic pain may lead to increases in neuroticism.

Two types of methodology have been used in trying to differentiate between psychopathology as a cause or consequence of headaches. One line of research has attempted to document changes in personality functioning as a result of treatment. Sovak, Kunzel, Sternbach, and Dalessio (1981), for example, reported that following headache treatment with biofeedback or medication, neuroticism significantly decreased in the clinically improved biofeedback group but remained unchanged in the clinically unimproved biofeedback and medication, as well as medication-improved groups. The authors interpreted their findings as suggesting that neuroticism is an integral part of migraine etiology rather than a result of chronic pain. Drawing etiological inferences from treatment studies is a dubious strategy, however.

The other research approach that has been used is a cross-sectional design in which headache sufferers of varying headache chronicity are compared on personality measures. The logic of this design is that if individuals who have had headaches for long periods are no more psychologically distressed than individuals who have had headaches for short periods, the implication is that psychopathology is a cause of headaches rather than vice versa. Arena, Andrasik, and Blanchard (1985) compared headache sufferers divided into three groups on the basis of percentage of life with headaches in terms of a comprehensive battery of psychological tests. Results indicated no significant differences between the groups. The authors noted, with appropriate caution, that one interpretation of the results was that the personality traits often found in headache sufferers are not a result of the pain experience but in fact were present before the pain problem started.

A more recent study by this group using a similar design claimed to find no support for the hypothesis that headaches cause psychopathology but modest support for the hypothesis that psychopathology causes headaches (Blanchard, Kirsch, Appelbaum, & Jaccard, 1989). The authors of this study went on to suggest that their data fit what they called an Initial Distress and Gradual Adjustment Model. Specifically, subjects appeared to have their highest levels of psychological distress early in their headache career (the first 3 years, particularly year 1), regardless of age of onset, and then gradually adjusted to it as they learned adaptive coping strategies. There was also a suggestion in the data that individuals with headaches of long duration showed a slight increase in psychological distress after 20 years.

Standing back from the literature, it seems likely that personality traits or profiles would act as predisposing factors for some types of headaches (e.g., headaches precipitated by stress) but not for others (e.g., headaches precipitated by perceptual stimuli). Also, it seems likely that a personality predisposition could take on a number of different forms rather than a single form. If these speculations have any validity, the search for a headache personality is misguided and researchers should adopt a different approach to investigating the relationship between personality and headaches.

Two recent studies are consistent with this argument. Following investigations that have demonstrated homogeneous subgroups in the chronic pain population (Sternbach, 1974; Bradley, Prokop, Margolis, & Gentry, 1978), Rappoport, McAnulty, Waggoner, and Brantely (1987) cluster-analyzed the MMPI profiles of a sample of 123 chronic headache sufferers recruited by advertisements. This resulted in four homogeneous subgroups characterized by (1) lack of significant elevations on any scale ($n = 54$), (2) relatively high but not clinically significant scores on scales 1, 2, and 3 ($n = 35$), (3) conversion V ($n = 18$), and (4) clinically significant elevations on scales 1,2,3,4 (Psychopathic Deviate, or anger), 6 (Paranoia), 7 (Psychasthenia, or anxiety), and 8 (Schizophrenia) ($n = 16$). A multiple discriminant analysis successfully classified 97.6% of the headache subjects to one of the four clusters. The obtained clusters closely resembled those found in previous pain research.

Robinson, Geisser, Dieter, and Swerdlow (1991) replicated the results of Rappoport et al. (1987) with a larger sample. The results of the two studies only differed in that Robinson et al. (1991) also identified a subgroup characterized by depression.

The results of these two studies clarify why the headache personality has proved so elusive: Chronic headache sufferers are not a homogeneous group with respect to personality characteristics. Overall, headache patients may demonstrate a conversion V or be characterized as neurotic, but this is due to elevated scores in a subset of the population. The data show that the subgroup characterized by lack of significant elevation on any scale comprised 44% (Rappaport et al., 1987) and 25% (Robinson et al., 1991) of the samples studied, and the subgroup characterized by relatively high but not clinically significant scores comprised 28% (Rappaport et al., 1987) and 37% (Robinson et al., 1991) of the samples studied. It seems likely that personality is not a predisposing factor for headaches in the first subgroup and perhaps not for the second subgroup but may be significant for the other subgroups.

Consequences

Immediate Reactions

The literature relevant to the immediate responses to headaches of sufferers and significant others will be reviewed according to the five hypotheses discussed in Chapter 1, although the hypotheses and related evidence do overlap.

REINFORCEMENT HYPOTHESIS

A number of writers who have advocated assessing headaches from a functional perspective have stressed the importance of focusing on the consequences of headaches (Lake, 1981; Norton & Nielson, 1977; Scott, 1979). Many others have argued that secondary gain plays an important role in a proportion of cases. M. J. Martin has expressed this view in several publications and suggested that headaches are a socially acceptable sign of distress that can be used for eliciting a show of concern and affection from family, friends, and physicians (Martin, M. J., 1983). He has suggested that some patients learn early in their headache career that they can escape their responsibilities and often literally control their environment (Martin, 1966).

Martin (1972) claimed to find evidence that such secondary gains were maintaining headache complaints in 56% of a sample of 100 headache sufferers. In a similar vein, Stout (1984) reported that 50% of a small migraine sample responded affirmatively to a secondary gain question (Does anything good or pleasant ever result from your migraine problem), and Packard, Andrasik, and Weaver (1989) discuss three cases of patients with migraine who often referred to their headaches as "good." Other authors have suggested that reinforcement for headache complaints is only likely to be of significance for a small minority of recurrent headache sufferers (Holroyd & Andrasik, 1982; Haynes, 1981).

Ehde, Holm, and Metzger (1991) found that migraine sufferers as compared to headache-free controls were more likely to describe their families as emphasizing clear organization, structure, rules, and overall control, but less likely to encourage emotional expression. They hypothesized that when emotionally expressive behaviors are not encouraged or accepted by the family, pain behaviors may substitute as an acceptable means of eliciting support and attention from family members. Therefore, pain behaviors may come to be reinforced in these families as acceptable ways to express emotional distress.

Unfortunately, no direct tests of the reinforcement hypothesis of headaches have been published but some indirect evidence is available. In one of my studies (Martin, Milech, & Nathan, 1992), factor analysis revealed that the most common pattern of responses to headaches by sufferers was to stop what they were doing and sit or lie down and take medication. The most common response pattern of partners to headaches was to offer sympathy, get medication, and encourage sufferers to stop what they were doing and sit or lie down. A response pattern by partners of encouraging sufferers to keep going, ignoring the headaches, complaining about the headaches, and lacking sympathy was a relatively rare reaction. Also, the findings showed a degree of synchrony between the reactions of sufferers and partners as, for example, sufferers who responded to headaches by eating and drinking reported that their partners tended to respond to headaches by getting them food and drink. Of course, these data do not demonstrate that headaches are maintained by their consequences but they are certainly consistent with this hypothesis. The data do emphasize that partners generally react to headaches in positive and supportive ways.

Other indirect evidence that relates to the reinforcement hypothesis comes from case studies using contingency management procedures. Yen and McIntire (1971) treated a 14-year-old girl with a response–cost approach that involved requiring the girl to write down information pertaining to her headaches before complaining about them or asking for medication. The aim was not to eliminate complaints or medication requests, because these behaviors could be adaptive, but to reduce their frequency. This "operant therapy" approach was successful in achieving these objectives. Ramsden, Friedman, and Williamson (1983) applied a contingency management procedure for the treatment of a 6-year-old female migraineur using a multiple-baseline-across-settings design. The results indicated a substantial reduction in reported headache pain over the 18 weeks of the study with continued maintenance of effects at a 10-month follow-up assessment. As noted earlier, however, treatment studies tend not to provide convincing data with respect to etiological mechanisms.

More evidence exists with respect to the role of reinforcement in other pain problems. Flor, Kerns, and Turk (1987), for example, reported a multiple regression analysis that revealed that spousal reinforcement of overt expressions of pain was significantly related to perceived pain in a mixed group of chronic pain sufferers (none with headache). Also, numerous papers have reported the successful application of operant approaches to the treatment of low back pain (e.g., Fordyce et al., 1973; Fordyce, 1976). It has been argued that the in-patient contingency management methods used with low back pain and other chronic pain problems are equally applicable to chronic headaches (Fowler, 1975), but data to support this claim have not been forthcoming.

AVOIDANCE BEHAVIOR HYPOTHESIS

Philips (1987a) has argued that avoidance behavior plays a role in maintaining chronic pain via increased sensitivity to pain-inducing stimuli in the short term and through adversely affecting self-efficacy beliefs pertaining to pain in the long term. This model is based on a number of different types of evidence, one of which is the data showing that a characteristic response to pain is avoidance behavior. Philips and Hunter (1981) developed a Pain Behavior Checklist (PBC) with 19 items divided into three categories (avoidance, complaints, and miscellaneous) and administered it to a sample of headache sufferers. They found that a number of the avoidance and complaint items were endorsed frequently by both tension headache and migraine sufferers. The correlation between avoidance and complaint items was low and neither of these forms of behavior was related to medication taking. Discordance was found when the behaviors from the PBC were related to the average intensity, frequency, and duration of the headache problem.

Since this paper was written, a number of studies have been reported in which the authors have administered versions of the PBC and factor-analyzed the results. Three factors emerged from an investigation by Anciano (1986): Avoidance, Verbal Complaint, and Palliative Behavior. Appelbaum, Radnitz, Blanchard, and Prins (1988) identified four factors: Avoidance, Verbal Complaint, Nonverbal Complaint, and Medication Consumption. Scores on all four factors were significantly positively correlated with anxiety and similarly for depression with the exception of the Verbal Complaint factor.

Philips and Jahanshahi (1986) extended the PBC to 49 items and administered it to a larger group of headache sufferers. The results did not confirm the hypothesized three components (avoidance, complaint, and help seeking) but showed a more complex structure consisting of 13 independent factors of pain behavior. Six avoidance factors emerged that accounted for 43% of the variance, the strongest of which was social avoidance or withdrawal, which accounted for 22% of the variance. High avoidance was associated with elevated depression.

Another type of evidence that supports Philips's model comes from one of her studies in which she investigated the functional significance of avoidance behavior in chronic pain (Philips & Jahanshahi, 1985). These authors proposed that exposure to a salient pain-provoking stimulus would lead to increasing tolerance by a process of adaptation, while avoidance of the stimulus would increase the potency of such stimuli to provoke pain. To test these predictions, a sample of chronic headache sufferers was exposed to noise stress. Results were in line with predictions and showed that exposure under optimal conditions (relaxation) was effective in reducing pain behaviors whereas avoidance of exposure to potent stimuli led to increasing intolerance.

Other evidence demonstrates that the increasing chronicity of headaches is associated with increasing avoidance behavior even though the severity of the pain problem does not appear to increase in parallel (Philips & Jahanshahi, 1985, 1986). Philips (1987a) goes on to argue that with the growth of avoidance behavior, there is evidence that patients report decreasing self-control of pain, and she cites one of her studies in support of this contention which found a high negative correlation between avoidance behaviors and self-efficacy beliefs (Philips, 1987b).

A second model of chronic pain focusing on avoidance behavior by Lethem et al. (1983) was outlined briefly in Chapter 1. Slade, Troup, Lethem, and Bentley (1983) collected data that they argued was in line with this model, but these data will not be discussed here because the study focused on low back pain and utilized a student sample. Headache sufferers showed greater fear of severe pain and less fear of minor pain compared to controls in a study by Hursey and Jacks (1992), which provided mixed support for the model since the former finding was in conflict with the model but the latter finding supported the model.

The studies reviewed in this section are clearly also relevant to the reinforcement hypothesis. For example, the finding of avoidance behavior in response to chronic pain is consistent with the suggestion that negative reinforcement plays a role in the maintenance of headaches. The finding of verbal and nonverbal complaints establishes the necessary conditions for social reinforcement because such behaviors ensure that other individuals in their vicinity realize that the sufferers are experiencing a headache.

EXACERBATING ANTECEDENTS HYPOTHESIS

Because there are many different antecedents of headaches, there are potentially many reactions to headaches that may stimulate the antecedents. This may occur via a vicious cycle involving stress and negative affect on the one hand and headaches on the other. Evidence was reviewed in the antecedents section that suggested a relationship between these two sets of variables. Most of the evidence did not distinguish among stress and negative affect causing headaches, the reverse direction relationship, or a reciprocal relationship.

Other studies have suggested that headaches result in distress and negative affect. Penzien, Holroyd, Holm, and Hursey (1985) administered to a sample of headache sufferers a 48-item scale developed by Bakal (1982) for assessing thoughts or feelings experienced at headache onset (Headache Assessment Questionnaire [HAQ]). Principal-components analysis of the data revealed four interpretable factors: Nonproductive Rumination, Self-denigration, Irritation over Environmental Difficulties, and Tension or Worry. For frequent headache sufferers, the HAQ was significantly correlated with headache activity indices, suggesting that people who experience more frequent and severe headaches also tend to experience more dysfunctional thoughts and negative affect.

Philips (1989) modified the HAQ in order to make it appropriate for any type of chronic pain, calling the revised version the Cognitive Evaluation Questionnaire (CEQ). The CEQ was then administered to a group of 72 back pain sufferers and 26 headache cases. An exploratory cluster analysis resulted in seven clusters: positive coping, desire to withdraw, disappointment with self, causal rumination, helplessness, concern with effects of pain, and emotional reactivity. Hence, with the exception of positive coping, the remaining six clusters emphasized the maladaptive nature of the majority of cognitive reactions associated with continuing or incrementing pain experience. Although these clusters are different from the factors found by Penzien et al. (1985), the results confirm the heterogeneity of pain cognitions, the majority of which are likely to play a role in enhancing or perpetuating chronic pain. Philips also pointed out how these data lend support to her avoidance model, as some of the identified clusters seem likely to play a role in motivating and/or maintaining the avoidance behavior characteristic of chronic pain sufferers.

Demjen, Bakal, and Dunn (1990) developed the 35-item Headache Cognitions Questionnaire to assess thoughts and feelings that commonly occur immediately before and during headache attacks. Principal-components analysis of the responses of headache sufferers to this questionnaire yielded two factors: headache-related distressing thoughts and feelings and situation-related distressing thoughts and feelings. Demjen et al. (1990) interpreted these data as supporting their hypothesis that headache disorders of increased severity are accompanied by a cognitive shift whereby the patient's primary concern moves from situational and interpersonal distress to distress associated with the disorder itself.

ENHANCING PAIN PERCEPTION HYPOTHESIS

In reviewing the literature on the psychology of pain, Melzack and Wall (1988) delineate a number of factors that affect pain perception. Elevations in anxiety have been shown to raise the intensity of perceived pain. Focusing attention on painful experiences has a similar effect. Finally, it has been demonstrated that if people feel they have control over their pain, the level of perceived pain is reduced even if they do not have control.

These findings seem relevant for chronic headache sufferers given some of the evidence reviewed so far. With respect to anxiety, a number of studies have been discussed that document an association between headaches and anxiety. With respect to whether headache sufferers focus on their headaches or distract themselves from the pain, the studies on cognitive reactions to pain reviewed in the previous section suggest that the predominant response is the former. Demjen et al. (1990) argue for a cognitive shift occurring with head pain of increased severity from situational interpersonal distress to distress associated with the headache. All the factors identified by Penzien et al. (1985) involved headaches, including one that consisted of ruminating about headaches. The seven clusters revealed by Philips (1989) all involved pain, including one ruminating about the causes of the pain and another on concern about the effects of the pain.

Sense of control over pain is an important feature of the avoidance model of chronic pain (Philips, 1987a). Philips argued that increased chronicity of pain is associated with increased avoidance behavior, and decreased feelings of self-control are a long-term effect of suffering from chronic headaches. Also, the study of Philips (1989) identified one of the cognitive reactions to pain as helplessness.

DRUG-INDUCED HYPOTHESIS

A common response to a headache's developing, or even to concern that a headache will develop, is to take medication, sometimes in large quantities. Wilkinson (1988) reported a case of a migraineur who consumed 315 tablets of antimigraine and other medications per week. Ergotamine tartrate has for the past 50 years been considered the drug of first choice for the treatment of acute migraine attacks, and analgesics are also considered useful for managing headaches (e.g., Saper, 1987; Baumgartner, Wessely, Bingol, Maly, & Holzner, 1989). Evidence is accumulating, however, that headaches can be induced by chronic substance abuse. This is recognized in the IHS classification system which includes the subcategories "ergotamine-induced headache" and "analgesic abuse headache." Baumgartner et al. (1989) claim that drug-induced headaches are a common problem, accounting for 10–15% of patients in headache clinics and about 1% of the general population.

It has been suggested that the daily ingestion of ergotamine may be a factor in converting migraine into chronic daily headache, and that ceasing medication may produce a corresponding improvement (Rowsell, Neylan, & Wilkinson, 1973). In a review of the ergotamine-induced headache literature, Saper (1987) concluded that when usage of ergotamine exceeds 2 or 3 days per week, it can result in a state of psychological and physiological dependency that appears to promote increasing usage of the drug and daily or almost daily headaches of a migraine type. Withholding the drug is characterized by intensification of the headache and associated symptoms during the period 12 to 72 hours following discontinuance.

Whether analgesic abuse can cause headaches is a subject of debate in the medical literature, with some authors arguing for (e.g., Baumgartner et al., 1989; Rapoport, 1988) and others against (e.g., Fisher, 1988; Bowdler, Kilian, & Gansslen-Blumberg, 1988). Lance, Parkes, and Wilkinson (1988) compared high and low analgesic users in a sample of nonmigrainous patients with chronic pain and found no significant differences between these two groups in terms of headache frequency. They concluded that analgesic abuse headaches may be restricted to those patients who are already sufferers.

A number of studies have reported headache improvement associated with analgesic withdrawal, although the discontinuation of medication has usually been accompanied by other treatment strategies rendering interpretation of results problematic. Rapoport, Weeks, Sheftell, Baskin, and Verdi (1985) studied the question of analgesic rebound headache in patients who had daily headaches and were consuming 14 or more analgesic tablets per week. Sixty-six percent of the sample improved considerably 1 month after discontinuing their analgesics and 81% were significantly improved at the end of the second month.

Baumgartner et al. (1989) reported good results associated with analgesic withdrawal in a chronic headache sample, but patients received additional treatment of both a pharmacological and psychological nature so that the specific effect of analgesic withdrawal was not determined. Mathew, Kurman, and Perez (1990) conducted a treatment study that involved manipulation of medication plus other forms of treatment (dietary advice and biofeedback training). They concluded that the daily use of symptomatic- or immediate-relief medications, which included ergotamine, analgesics, and other medications, resulted in chronic daily headaches. They also reported that discontinuance of daily symptomatic medications resulted in headache improvement.

Long-Term Effects

Some of the long-term effects of headaches have already been discussed, (e.g., decreased self-efficacy with respect to control of pain). Associations documented in the antecedents section between headaches on the one hand and personality characteristics, psychopathology, and social support on the other may reflect the consequences of headaches rather than, or as well as, the causes of headaches.

An early study that included data on the long-term effects of headaches was carried out by Barnat and Lake (1983). These authors devised an attitudes survey and administered it to patients attending a headache clinic. Findings included that 50% felt that headaches interrupted their daily routine much or all of the time. Forty-one percent believed that headaches prevented problem solving, and 28% believed that if their headaches went away, most of their problems would be solved. Sixty-four percent considered that their life would be richer without headaches.

Lacroix and Barbaree (1990) administered a shortened version of the Comprehensive Pain Questionnaire (CPQ) to a headache sample recruited through a combination of physician referral, media advertisements, and undergraduate classes. Questions on the CPQ have been divided into three categories: (1) impact on life-style, (2) impact on general health, (3) overall appraisal of headache impact. With respect to life-style, 65% of respondents indicated that headaches affected their ability to carry out their occupation. Thirty-two percent reported experiencing decreased satisfaction with their work and 20% found that the headaches interfered with their ability to get along with coworkers. A job change was necessary because of the pain for 17% of the sample. Twenty-one percent reported having discontinued specific leisure activities as a result of their headaches and 26% reported making changes in their social life. Changes on both these variables were reported much more frequently by women than by men.

With respect to impact on general health, 51% reported having changed their sleep habits since the onset of their headaches. Sleep problems were fairly evenly divided between difficulty falling asleep, waking during the night, and early-morning waking. Women consistently reported more sleep problems. Twenty-three percent indicated that their weight had changed significantly since the headache started.

Overall, 54% reported headaches to be a very serious problem, a high figure considering the method of recruiting the sample.

Two recent papers have reported the results of administering the Nottingham Health Profile (NHP) to a migraine sample. The NHP purports to measure perceived health status via scores on six domains: energy, pain, emotional reactions, sleep, social isolation, and physical mobility (Jenkinson, 1990; Jenkinson & Fitzpatrick, 1990). The migraineurs' scores were higher than the normative values on all domains except pain and mobility. The absence of an elevated score on the pain scale was a curious feeling. The authors interpreted their results as emphasizing the psychosocial consequences of migraine and the impact it has on the life of sufferers.

Carlsson, Augustinsson, Blomstrand, and Sullivan (1990) administered the Sickness Impact Profile to a tension headache sample. This questionnaire measures health status via scores on 12 categories. Comparison of the headache group to a general population reference group indicated greater "sickness impact" on the overall scores, three of the four psychosocial categories (emotional behavior, social interaction, and alertness behavior) and three of the five independent categories (work, sleep and rest, home management), but none of the three physical categories.

The stress of living with certain types of headaches was suggested by the recent findings of Breslau and her colleagues (Breslau, Davis, & Andreski, 1991; Breslau, 1992). They reported an association between migraine with aura and suicidal ideation and suicide attempts, a relationship that held up even when depression was controlled for.

Summary

The evidence reviewed in this chapter makes a strong case for a link between stress and negative affect and headaches. The onset of headaches is often associated with stressful events. Headaches flourish when life-style or life situation is characterized by stress and negative emotion. And most important, headaches often begin or become more intense in response to stress and negative affect. The evidence for stress and negative feelings as precipitants of headaches comes from several sources. Stress and negative affect are the most frequently reported triggers for headaches, studies employing self-monitoring have demonstrated that they commonly occur in conjunction with headaches, and manipulations of stress and mood have resulted in changes in headache activity. Our understanding of the relationship between stress and headaches has been enhanced by studies suggesting that headache sufferers in comparison to nonheadache controls experience more daily hassles and possibly more life-event stress, appraise stressful events more negatively, employ less effective coping strategies, and perceive themselves as having less social support available.

It would be a mistake to overemphasize the strength of the relationship between stress and negative affect and headaches, however. Not all headache onsets are associated with stress. Reported correlations between stress and negative affect and headaches have usually been of low magnitude, and where analyses have focused on individuals, large differences have been found with very strong relationships for some individuals and no relationship for others.

The evidence pertaining to the relationship between food and headaches is mixed. Some studies have found that food is a commonly reported precipitant but others have not. Prospective studies have yielded support for a relationship between food and headaches. Comparison of consumption of chocolate, the most commonly reported dietary trigger of headaches, and placebo did not support the role of chocolate as an inducer of headaches, but a similar trial with aspartame yielded positive findings. A controlled trial manipulating diet in a standardized way failed to show any significant effect of diet, but a number of studies treating headaches via individualized (elimination) diets have produced impressive results. Support for the importance of fasting as a precipitating factor comes from retrospective surveys, prospective studies, and manipulation studies.

It has been suggested that hormonally mediated factors such as menarche and use of oral contraceptives are implicated in the onset of some headaches in women. Also, it is argued that the phase of the menstrual cycle may act as a setting factor for headaches or may directly precipitate headaches. Many other factors have been suggested as capable of precipitating or aggravating headaches, including perceptual stimuli (e.g., flicker, glare, noise) and seasonal and meteorological conditions (e.g., change of weather, heat, humidity). The evidence to support these associations is largely limited to patients' retrospective self-report, however, so the validity of such claims remains to be tested empirically.

There is a tendency for headaches to run in families and genetic factors seem to play a role. Heredity appears to be less important than was believed to be the case in the past, however. Whether transmission is through a dominant gene, a recessive gene, or numerous genes remains unclear.

The extensive literature on headaches and personality does not support the clinically derived concept of a migraine or headache personality. The evidence does suggest that overall, chronic sufferers are more psychologically distressed and have more deviant personality characteristics than do nonheadache sufferers. Even this statement needs to be qualified, however, as the findings supporting this conclusion may be an artifact of subject selection reflecting the biased sample who visit clinicians or volunteer for research, or an artifact of the personality inventories measuring headache symptomatology rather than psychopathology. Also, there is some doubt as to whether the personality characteristics associated with headaches are unique to headaches or associated with a variety of psychosomatic disorders. A final interpretive problem concerns whether the observed psychopathology is a cause, consequence, or concomitant of chronic headaches, although studies that have addressed this issue suggest that psychopathology precedes headaches. Recent research suggests that a number of homogeneous subgroups can be identified in the headache population some of which are characterized by deviant personality characteristics and some of which are not.

Surprisingly little research has been carried out on the consequences of headaches. The review of literature relevant to immediate reactions to headaches was organized according to five hypotheses relating to how responses to headaches might be maladaptive. For each hypothesis, it was possible to cite some evidence that was consistent with it, but the support was generally indirect and inconclusive.

Whereas headaches are a distressing experience for the sufferer, they are often followed by events that appear likely to be reinforcing, although whether this serves to increase the probability of further headaches is uncertain. Behavioral reactions to headaches are characterized by avoidance, verbal complaints, nonverbal complaints, and medication consumption. Cognitive reactions to headaches are dominated by negative thoughts involving rumination, self-denigration, worry, and irritation over environmental difficulties. Affective reactions are characterized by a range of negative emotions.

Over the long term, headaches result in cognitive changes, including decreased feelings of self-efficacy with respect to control of pain. Headaches impact on life-style, for example, affecting ability to carry out occupational demands and leading to discontinuance of leisure activities and changes in social life. Headaches affect other areas of functioning—most notably sleep. Some consequences associated with headaches seem greater for women than for men, which may partially explain why women disproportionately consult doctors and volunteer for research studies.

5

Studies of Psychological Treatment of Headaches

The main focus of psychological research on headaches has been on treatment studies. This extensive literature will be organized in 10 sections. The first eight consider different treatment modalities, starting with clinic-based programs administered on an individual basis. Most outcome data from treatment studies pertain to headache parameters, but the ninth section considers the effects of treatment programs on other variables. The final section discusses predictors of improvement and data pertaining to client-treatment matching.

For each type of treatment discussed, the following issues will be considered: the nature of the treatment and its rationale, treatment efficacy (i.e., how it compares to control conditions such as no treatment and attention–placebo), comparative efficacy (i.e., how it compares to alternative treatments), percentage of success, maintenance of treatment gains, and mechanisms of change. It should be emphasized, however, that relevant data are not available for all these issues for all treatments.

Before beginning the review, a few comments about terminology are necessary. Different names have been used by various writers for the same or substantially similar treatment techniques. In this review, consistent terminology will be used even when this results in departures from the original labels provided by the authors. The term *thermal biofeedback* will be used to cover all forms of thermal and temperature biofeedback; *BVP biofeedback* will be used to include pulse amplitude biofeedback, vasomotor biofeedback, and vasoconstriction training; and *cognitive coping training* will be used to include cognitive therapy, cognitive–behavioral treatment, stress-coping training, and cognitive skills training.

Clinic-based individually administered treatment has typically involved approximately 10 sessions (Holroyd & Penzien, 1986). The impact of treatment on headaches is almost invariably evaluated via patients' self-monitoring of headache activity on an hourly or four-times-a-day basis (see Chapter 6 for a fuller discussion of self-monitoring headaches). Other pain measures are sometimes also included for pre- to posttreatment comparisons of which the most common is the McGill Pain Questionnaire (Melzack, 1975). A variety of measures have been derived from "headache diaries," including headache frequency, average headache intensity, average headache duration, percentage of headache-free days, and peak headache intensity, although the most common is a composite headache index comprising the average intensity rating. A small minority of studies have reported differential treatment effects on alternative pain measures, but no consistent pattern has emerged, and this review does not differentiate between the different measures.

EMG Biofeedback Training

EMG biofeedback training involves providing patients with continuous information pertaining to the state of tension of one or more muscles with a view to helping them control the tension. The muscle site most commonly used in the treatment of headaches has been the forehead, but some studies have given feedback from the neck muscles (Martin & Mathews, 1978; Otis, Turner, & Low, 1975) and others from the muscle showing the highest resting EMG level (Peck & Kraft, 1977; Philips, 1977c). The laboratory training has generally been accompanied by instructions to practice relaxing at home each day, but there have been exceptions (e.g., Epstein, Hersen, & Hemphill, 1974; Kondo & Canter, 1977). EMG biofeedback training has often been combined with relaxation training.

This form of biofeedback training has mainly been used with tension headache sufferers, and the rationale with this group is obvious given that such headaches are allegedly caused by stress leading to excessive tension in pericranial muscles. However, EMG biofeedback training has also been used with migraineurs (e.g., Bakal & Kaganov, 1977; Lake, Rainey, & Papsdorf, 1979), for which a number of rationales have been offered: (1) migraines are often precipitated or aggravated by stress and tension, (2) the physiological mechanism of migraine may include a muscular component, and (3) EMG biofeedback can serve as an attention–placebo control procedure for treatments targeted at relevant (i.e., vascular) mechanisms.

Numerous studies have shown EMG biofeedback training to be superior to a headache monitoring (i.e., no-treatment) control condition for reducing tension headaches (e.g., Haynes et al., 1975; Chesney & Shelton, 1976). Other studies have demonstrated EMG biofeedback to be superior to a variety of attention–placebo control procedures such as "pseudofeedback" (e.g., Budzynski, Stoyva, Adler, & Mullaney, 1973; Philips, 1977c) and "medication placebo" (Cox, Freundlich, & Meyer, 1975). These control conditions look less than satisfactory, however, because procedures such as pseudofeedback (recording of successful EMG feedback session played to patients who were told it was a monotonous tone that would help them relax) and medication placebo (patients given a glucose tablet that they were told would help them relax) seem unlikely to raise expectations of success to the same level as EMG biofeedback training, which has considerable face validity. A study by Holroyd, Andrasik, and Noble (1980), however, demonstrated that EMG biofeedback training was significantly superior to a pseudotherapy condition ("meditation") which had been rated by subjects as equally credible as the EMG biofeedback training.

Many studies have compared EMG biofeedback training with relaxation training and most have found them to be equally effective (e.g., Cox et al., 1975; Martin & Mathews, 1978). Hutchings and Reinking (1976), however, found EMG biofeedback and relaxation training to be equally superior to relaxation training alone, and Chesney and Shelton (1976) found relaxation training and the combination of EMG biofeedback and relaxation training to be equally more effective than EMG biofeedback alone. Blanchard, Andrasik, Neff, Arena et al. (1982) showed that EMG biofeedback training led to further significant reductions in headache activity in tension headache sufferers who failed to respond to relaxation training.

Other treatments have been compared with EMG biofeedback training and in almost all cases they have been shown to be equally effective: transcendental meditation (Winkler, 1979), hypnotic analgesia (Schlutter, Golden, & Blume, 1980); thermal biofeedback training (Daly, Donn, Galliher, & Zimmerman, 1983), and EEG biofeedback training and BVP biofeedback training (Cohen, McArthur, & Rickles, 1980). One exception is a study by Holroyd et al. (1977) that demonstrated that cognitive coping training was significantly more effective than EMG biofeedback training. The results of this study are difficult to interpret, however, as subjects in the biofeedback condition showed much less improvement than has been attained in most other studies, a result that Holroyd et al. suggest may have arisen from the use of "counterdemand" instructions (subjects were told that no improvement could be expected until the completion of treatment).

Blanchard, Andrasik, Ahles, Teders, and O'Keefe (1980) carried out a meta-analysis of all studies evaluating EMG biofeedback training and relaxation training for tension headache sufferers. These authors concluded that forehead EMG biofeedback, relaxation training, and a combination of these two procedures were equally effective and significantly superior to psychological placebo, medication placebo, and headache monitoring only. The average percentage of improvement associated with these six conditions was 60.9%, 59.2%, 58.8%, 35.3%, 34.8%, and −4.5%, respectively. A more recent meta-analysis produced similar findings in that EMG biofeedback, relaxation training, and a combination of the two were equally effective and all superior to noncontingent feedback and headache monitoring (Holroyd & Penzien, 1986). This review resulted in lower percentage improvement figures, however, with findings of 46%, 44.6%, 57.1%, 15.3%, and −3.9%, respectively.

Blanchard (1987) reviewed 10 reports of prospective follow-ups of at least 12 month's duration for psychological treatments of chronic headaches. He concluded that the reduction in tension headaches obtained with forehead EMG biofeedback training deteriorated progressively at 2 and 3 years but not back to pretreatment levels.

With respect to mechanisms of change, the available evidence suggests that treatment gains associated with EMG biofeedback training are more than just a placebo effect. Some studies have reported positive correlations between reduction in EMG activity and headache improvement (e.g., Budzynski et al., 1973; Cox et al., 1975), and this supports the treatment rationale of learned control of physiological processes, but other studies have failed to find significant correlations (e.g., Epstein & Abel, 1977; Martin & Mathews, 1978).

To clarify the relationship between changes in EMG activity and headaches, Andrasik and Holroyd (1980a) directly manipulated the former in three biofeedback conditions. All groups were instructed similarly and were led to believe that they were learning to reduce forehead EMG, but in fact training focused on teaching subjects to decrease, increase, or hold stable forehead EMG. Results indicated that while EMG levels shifted in the intended directions, the headaches of the three biofeedback groups all improved significantly and equally. These findings were interpreted as suggesting that biofeedback works because subjects are implicitly encouraged to alter the cognitive and behavioral responses to headache-eliciting situations.

Holroyd et al. (1984) extended this model in an experiment in which subjects were assigned to one of four conditions: increase or decrease EMG (as in their earlier study) and high-success feedback or low-success feedback (achieved via bogus video displays). The authors reported that regardless of actual changes in EMG activity, subjects receiving high-success feedback showed substantially greater improvement in headache activity (53%) than did subjects receiving moderate-success feedback (26%). Performance feedback was also found to be related to changes in locus of control and self-efficacy, and changes in these two cognitive variables during biofeedback training were also correlated with reduction in headache activity following treatment. These results have led the authors to devise a new model of therapeutic change in which it is hypothesized as follows:

> [I]f patients perceive biofeedback training as a credible treatment and perceive themselves as succeeding at the biofeedback task through their own efforts, they

will view (a) their headaches as having an internal locus of control, and (b) themselves as self-efficacious (i.e., as capable of influencing their headaches). These cognitive changes are expected to lead to new and more persistent efforts to cope with headache-related stresses that, in turn, alter psychological and physiological stress-responses triggering headaches. (p. 1040)

Thermal Biofeedback Training

Thermal biofeedback training involves providing subjects with continuous information pertaining to skin temperature. In the original application of this approach to migraine, feedback was provided of the differential temperature between the mid-forehead and the right index finger (Sargent, Green, & Walters, 1972) with the training goal of "warm hand, cool head." It was later found that the major temperature changes took place in the hands, resulting in researchers providing feedback from this site alone. Autogenic phases are usually introduced to assist the subject's efforts but not always (e.g., Reading & Mohr, 1976; Turin & Johnson, 1976), and subjects are generally encouraged to practice hand warming at home on a daily basis. Thermal biofeedback training has frequently been accompanied by relaxation training. A number of variations of this procedure have been investigated and they will be discussed at the end of this section.

With respect to treatment rationale, thermal biofeedback training was first introduced as a result of a serendipitous finding. A research subject at the Menninger Foundation demonstrated considerable flushing in her hands with an accompanying 10°F rise in 2 minutes during the spontaneous recovery from a migraine attack (Sargent, Green, & Walters, 1973). Knowledge of this event prompted two migraineurs to volunteer for training in hand temperature control. One was wholly successful and learned to eliminate migraine for the most part. The other had a partially beneficial result and she was able to alleviate headache intensity somewhat and reduce frequency of headaches (Sargent, Walters, & Green, 1973).

Thermal biofeedback training has mainly been used as a treatment for migraine, although it has also been used as a treatment for tension headache (Daly et al., 1983). Conflicting rationales for its use have been proposed. Elmore and Tursky (1981) argue that thermal biofeedback training leads to temporal vasodilation and hence is useful for preventing or aborting headaches as the preheadache phase is believed to be associated with vasoconstriction. This position is based on the belief that thermal biofeedback training produces a general reduction in autonomic arousal. In contrast, Knapp (1982) argues that thermal biofeedback training results in temporal vasoconstriction and hence is useful for countering the dilation of the extracranial vasculature that occurs during the headache phase.

A number of studies have demonstrated that thermal biofeedback training was superior to no treatment (e.g., Blanchard, Theobald, Williamson, Silver, & Brown, 1978; Gauthier et al., 1985). Two studies have compared thermal biofeedback training with a pseudofeedback condition to control for attention–placebo effects, and both reported that the true and false conditions were equally associated with reduction in headaches (Mullinix, Norton, Hack, & Fishman, 1978; Reading, 1984). A number of investigations have used thermal biofeedback training for hand cooling as an attention–placebo control condition for hand warming. Most of these studies found no differences in headache relief between the two conditions (e.g., Gauthier, Bois, Allaire, & Drolet, 1981; Largen, Mathew, Dobbins, & Claghorn, 1981), but two small studies have reported that hand cooling is associated with headache activity's remaining the same or increasing (Johnson & Turin, 1975; Turin & Johnson, 1976).

In addition to comparing hand warming and cooling, Gauthier et al. (1981) compared thermal biofeedback training from the finger versus a site over the temporal artery. The different sites did not lead to differential reductions in migraine activity. Blanchard, Appelbaum, Radnitz, Morrill et al. (1990) used pseudomeditation as an attention–placebo control condition and reported no significant differences between this procedure and two thermal biofeedback training conditions, although on a measure of clinically significant improvement the two biofeedback groups showed a higher degree of improvement (51.6%) than did the pseudomeditation group (37.5%).

The results of these studies suggest that thermal biofeedback training achieves its success via placebo mechanisms. There are a number of arguments against this interpretation, however. First, most of the studies reviewed have used small subject samples and hence lack statistical power to detect differences. This criticism particularly applies to the pseudofeedback studies, which both employed seven or less subjects per condition. Second, training hand cooling may be therapeutic as a result of psychophysiological processes. Gauthier et al. (1981), for example, have suggested that stabilization of peripheral vascular activity rather than a specific directional change such as hand warming is the therapeutic element. Alternatively, if stage theories of migraine involving both cranial vasoconstriction and vasodilation are accepted, both hand warming and hand cooling could be efficacious. Subjects would need to learn to apply the trained skills at different stages of the migraine cycle, depending on which type of training they received. Similarly, the pseudomeditation condition may have been therapeutic, since patients appeared to construe it as a form of relaxation training (Blanchard, Applebaum, Radnitz, Morrill et al., 1990).

Thermal biofeedback training has been compared with many other treatments and almost all such comparisons have failed to show significant differences. Null findings have been reported in comparisons with progressive relaxation training (Blanchard et al., 1978), EEG biofeedback training and training in self-hypnosis (Andreychuk & Skriver, 1975), forehead EMG biofeedback training and skin conductance biofeedback training (Reading, 1984), forehead EMG biofeedback training (Lake et al., 1979), forehead EMG biofeedback training and autogenic phrases (Sargent, Solbach, Coyne, Spohn, & Segerson, 1986), forehead EMG biofeedback training and progressive relaxation training (Daly et al., 1983), and BVP biofeedback training (Gauthier et al., 1985). Blanchard, Andrasik, Neff, Arena et al. (1982) showed that thermal biofeedback training led to further significant reductions in headache activity in migraineurs who failed to respond to relaxation training.

One exception to all the studies reporting nonsignificant findings is an investigation by Elmore and Tursky (1981) which found that BVP biofeedback training was significantly superior in reducing migraine activity to thermal biofeedback training. In this study, however, the thermal biofeedback condition was totally ineffective in contrast to the numerous studies reporting positive results with this approach. The significant findings of Elmore and Turksy for temporal constriction therefore parallel the significant findings of Holroyd et al. (1977) for cognitive coping training in that both studies seemed to achieve statistically significant differences by virtue of one treatment condition's attaining inferior results to those gained in other studies.

Blanchard et al. (1980) reported a meta-analytic comparison of thermal biofeedback training with autogenic training, thermal biofeedback training, relaxation training, and medication placebo in the treatment of migraine and found the three treatment conditions to be equally effective and significantly superior to medication placebo. Average improvement associated with the four conditions was 65.1%, 51.8%, 52.7%, and 16.5%, respectively. Holroyd and Penzien (1990) completed a meta-analytic review comparing thermal biofeedback training combined with relaxation training against pharmacological treatment (propranolol HCl) of migraine. Average improvement associated with these two treatment conditions, placebo and no treatment, was 55.1%, 55.1%, 12.2%, and 1.1%, respectively.

The review of long-term effects of psychological treatments referred to earlier concluded that there was good maintenance of headache reduction at 12 months for migraineurs treated with thermal biofeedback training (Blanchard, 1987). However, beyond 12 months there was tentative support for persistent, progressive deterioration, year by year, over a 4-year follow-up. A recent study reported more optimistic findings, as headache reductions achieved at the end of treatment persisted for up to 6 years and were in fact slightly enhanced during the follow-up period (Lisspers & Ost, 1990b). Also, Holroyd et al. (1989) followed-up migraineurs treated either with combined thermal biofeedback training and relaxation training or abortive pharmacological treatment (ergotamine tartrate). Patients in both treatment groups continued to show lower headache activity at 3-year follow-up than they had prior to treatment. Andrasik, Blanchard, Neff, and Rodichok (1984) found that booster sessions did not improve maintenance.

The mechanism of action of thermal biofeedback training is somewhat obscure. As noted earlier, directly contrasting rationales have been forwarded, and studies have been unable to conclusively demonstrate that this form of biofeedback training is significantly superior to appropriate attention–placebo control procedures. Any proposed mechanism has to take into account that hand cooling seems to be as effective for reducing headaches as hand warming is. Several studies have found no relationship between temperature control and headache changes (e.g., Gauthier et al., 1981; Mullinix et al., 1978).

A recent study by Morrill and Blanchard (1989) pursued the mechanism issue by investigating two hypotheses, the first of which was that a specific dose-response relationship existed such that subjects with greater physiological changes in the target response would evidence greater improvement in headache activity. This hypothesis received little support. The second hypothesis was that thermal biofeedback training has a much more generalized effect similar to relaxation training, which works by altering multiple autonomic nervous system responses. This hypothesis received stronger support. It was found that migraineurs who were treatment successes had significantly lowered their heart rates from pre- to posttreatment assessment. These findings were in line with an earlier study that demonstrated that thermal biofeedback training was not associated with the conditioning of a single response but was related to a general decrease in sympathetic tonic outflow with improvement of migraine activity (Dalessio, Kunzel, Sternbach, & Sovak, 1979).

An alternative possibility is that the critical changes induced by thermal biofeedback training are cognitive rather than physiological, as advocated by Holroyd et al. (1984) for EMG biofeedback training. This possibility received some support from a recent study by Mizener, Thomas, and Billings (1988) which showed that migraineurs treated with thermal biofeedback training became more internal about their beliefs to control their general health, held higher beliefs of ability to control their physiological processes, and were ignoring their pain sensations more than when they started treatment. There was a trend for patients to increase the use of coping self-statements and to decrease catastrophizing.

Variations on Thermal Biofeedback Training

Stout (1985) developed "homeostatic reconditioning" in which subjects learned to raise finger temperature after stressful imaginal exposure. Subjects trained in this vascular recovery after stress procedure tended to show more headache improvement than others who raised finger temperature following neutral imaginal exposure, but the differences were not significant.

Johansson and Ost (1987) added "generalization training" to thermal biofeedback training to enhance self-control in the absence of external feedback and application of skills in everyday life. The results of the study did not confirm that the additional training resulted in a higher degree of control of peripheral skin temperature or in greater migraine decrease.

Lake et al. (1979) added rational–emotive therapy (RET) to thermal biofeedback training. This did not significantly increase treatment efficacy, but the study included only six subjects in each condition. Blanchard, Appelbaum, Radnitz, Morrill et al. (1990) added cognitive coping training to thermal biofeedback training but found that the combination was no more effective than thermal biofeedback alone. As noted by the authors, however, the amount of time devoted to cognitive therapy in this study was very small, with total treatment time being extended by, on average, 25 minutes or 3.3%.

BVP Biofeedback Training

BVP biofeedback training involves providing subjects with continuous information with respect to pulse amplitude. In the treatment of headaches, the signal is recorded with some form of plethysmographic transducer positioned over the superficial temporal artery, usually on the side on which pain is experienced most frequently. The aim is for subjects to learn to decrease pulse amplitude, which is considered equivalent to constricting the artery, although it was argued in Chapter 3 that equating pulse amplitude with arterial diameter is a dubious assumption.

BVP biofeedback training has been used exclusively to treat migraine rather than other types of headaches except for some early case studies by Adams and colleagues (e.g., Feuerstein, Adams, & Beiman, 1976; Sturgis, Tollison, & Adams, 1978). The rationale of this form of biofeedback training is to teach subjects to voluntarily constrict the extracranial temporal artery, thereby countering the vasodilation associated with the head pain of migraine. Hence, this approach has been viewed as mimicking the action of the ergotamine derivatives that are traditionally used in the pharmacological treatment of migraine.

A number of studies have shown BVP biofeedback training to be significantly superior to headache monitoring (e.g., Bild & Adams, 1980; Gauthier et al., 1983). An early study that compared BVP biofeedback training with an attention–placebo control condition was carried out by Friar and Beatty (1976). These authors contrasted training in vasoconstriction of the extracranial arteries with training in vasoconstriction at an irrelevant site (the hand) and showed that the experimental condition was associated with a significant decrease in the incidence of major headache attacks, which was not so for the control condition. Bild and Adams (1980) compared BVP biofeedback training with an irrelevant treatment for migraine relief, namely, forehead EMG biofeedback training, and found the former to be significantly superior in reducing headache activity.

Gauthier et al. (1983) contrasted BVP biofeedback training in temporal artery constriction with training in temporal artery dilation. Results showed that these two conditions were equally effective in controlling migraines, but the authors argued against interpreting their findings as an indication that BVP biofeedback training is a mere placebo treatment. Their data showed that "reductions in migraine were . . . closely associated with reductions in the variability of the BVP response, thereby suggesting that voluntary vasoconstriction and vasodilation were effective because they both provided a physiological condition incompatible with extreme vasomotor activity" (p. 439).

Because it has been argued that the migraine cycle involves a pre-headache phase characterized by vasoconstriction and a headache phase characterized by vasodilation, Lisspers and Ost (1990a) suggested that training in both vasoconstriction and vasodilation could be therapeutic, with the self-regulation skills needing to be applied in different phases. These authors compared three conditions: (1) BVP biofeedback training in temporal artery constriction and instructions to apply these skills during headaches, (2) the same training and instructions to apply the skills between headaches (a condition expected to be ineffective), and (3) BVP biofeedback training to dilate the temporal arteries and instructions to use these skills during stress periods. The first group decreased their headaches by 58% at the end of treatment and by 68% at 6-month follow-up, while the other two groups decreased their headaches by 32% to 35% and 33% to 53%, respectively. The first group contained a significantly higher proportion of successful subjects than did the other two groups.

With respect to comparative efficacy, as discussed previously, Elmore and Tursky (1981) found BVP biofeedback training to be superior to thermal biofeedback training, but Gauthier et al. (1985) found no significant difference between these two conditions. Cohen et al. (1980) compared BVP biofeedback training with thermal biofeedback training (differential finger–forehead temperature), forehead EMG biofeedback training, and electroencephalogram (EEG) biofeedback training and found no significant differences between any of these conditions. Knapp and Florin (1981) assigned subjects to BVP biofeedback training, cognitive coping training, or a combination of the two. Each treatment condition was equally effective.

Data on the long-term maintenance of headache reduction achieved by BVP biofeedback training are very limited, but Lisspers and Ost (1990b) reported a 5-year follow-up of their earlier study (Lisspers & Ost, 1990a). They found very slight deterioration from their original 6-month follow-up to the long-term follow-up (from 56% to 48% reduction of the pretreatment levels). BVP biofeedback training did not significantly differ from thermal biofeedback training in terms of maintenance.

With respect to mechanisms of change, the balance of evidence suggests that BVP biofeedback training is more than a placebo treatment. Data relevant to the relationship between BVP self-regulation skills and headache reduction are inconsistent, however, with Gauthier et al. (1983) and Gauthier et al. (1985) reporting no significant relationship and Lisspers and Ost (1990a) reporting a significant relationship. Findings from the studies of Gauthier and his colleagues have been conflicting. One study found that headache improvement was associated with increased BVP variability (Gauthier et al., 1985) in contrast to an earlier study that found that improvement was associated with decreased BVP variability (Gauthier et al., 1983).

Falkenstein and Hoormann (1987) investigated the mechanism of BVP biofeedback training by monitoring a number of physiological variables during training. Parallel to BVP changes, the authors found heart rate acceleration, pulse transit time reduction (implying systolic blood pressure), and skin warming at the forehead. The authors interpret their findings as suggesting that learned sympathetic activation may account for a major part of the reduction in BVP amplitude, but that a second, related mechanism, regional arteriolar dilation, seems to be involved also, as arteriolar dilation leads to a reduction of peripheral resistance, which in turn causes BVP decrease.

Relaxation Training

Relaxation training as a treatment for headaches has usually been administered in the form of progressive relaxation training or autogenic training. Relaxation instructions are most commonly given "live" by a therapist but have occasionally been delivered by tape recorder. Relaxation training in the clinic is usually accompanied by instructions to practice at home on a daily basis.

Whereas the different forms of biofeedback training are generally used for particular types of headaches, relaxation training has been employed widely with both tension headaches and migraines. The two related rationales underlying relaxation training are that it combats the stress and tension that precipitates and aggravates both tension headaches and migraines and that it operates directly on the psychophysiological mechanisms (muscle tension for tension headaches; muscle tension or preheadache vasoconstriction for migraines).

Studies have shown relaxation training to be superior to no treatment for reducing headaches (Blanchard et al., 1978; Blanchard, Appelbaum, Radnitz, Michultka et al., 1990). Cox et al. (1975) demonstrated that relaxation training led to greater headache improvement than did medication placebo and Blanchard, Appelbaum, Radnitz, Michultka et al. (1990) demonstrated that relaxation training was more effective than an equally credible pseudomeditation attention–placebo control condition.

As reviewed in earlier sections of this chapter, most comparisons between relaxation training and EMG biofeedback training have suggested equal efficacy for decreasing headaches, and likewise for comparisons between relaxation training and thermal biofeedback training. Meta-analytic reviews have concluded that relaxation training was equally effective to these forms of biofeedback training and was significantly superior to placebo control conditions. These reviews produced improvement rates associated with relaxation training for tension headaches of 59.2% (Blanchard et al., 1980) and 44.6% (Holroyd & Penzien, 1986), and an improvement rate associated with relaxation training for migraines of 52.7% (Blanchard et al., 1980).

Sorbi and Tellegen (1986) investigated the differential efficacy of relaxation training and cognitive coping training in migraineurs. Both approaches led to significant reductions in migraine activity with no difference between the two, but there was a nonsignificant trend for cognitive coping training to be more effective at 8-month follow-up. Fin, DiGiuseppe, and Culver (1991) compared progressive relaxation and RET for the treatment of tension headaches and found both treatments to be equally superior to two control conditions ("headache discussion" and waiting list).

Blanchard, Appelbaum, Radnitz, Michultka et al. (1990) compared relaxation training with relaxation training plus cognitive coping training. Headache activity comparisons between the treatments showed no advantage to adding cognitive therapy to progressive relaxation training, but a measaure of clinically significant change showed a trend for the combination to be superior to relaxation alone. The authors concluded that adding cognitive coping training to relaxation training probably yields an advantage and clinically they would recommend this combination.

With respect to the long-term effects of relaxation training, the review by Blanchard (1987) concluded that for tension headache sufferers relief is maintained for at least 4 years, but for individuals with migraine or combined headaches progressive deterioration occurs after 12 months. On the other hand, a recent long-term study of relaxation training with migraineurs reported very good maintenance at 3-year follow-up (Sorbi, Tellegen, & Du Long, 1989).

With respect to mechanisms of change, the available evidence suggests that relaxation training is more than a placebo effect. Precisely how headache improvement is achieved is quite unclear, however.

Cognitive Coping Training

Two main variations of cognitive coping training have been developed. In the original formulation of this approach, Holroyd et al. (1977) focused on altering maladaptive cognitive responses that were assumed to mediate the occurrence of headaches. These authors offered a rationale in terms of headaches resulting from psychological stress with stress responses determined by cognitions about an event or situation. In contrast, Bakal, Demjen, and Kaganov (1981) developed a treatment approach that emphasized modifying stress reactions associated with headaches (feelings of helplessness, anxiety, fear) rather than modifying stress reactions to environmental and interpersonal events. They argued that this shift in emphasis from stress-coping skills to headache-coping skills was necessary because chronic headache sufferers experienced attacks in the absence of identifiable external or internal precipitants (see Chapter 4).

Cognitive coping training utilizes specific procedures adapted from various cognitive theorists, most notably Meichenbaum (e.g., Meichenbaum, 1977) and Beck (e.g., Beck, Rush, Shaw, & Emery, 1979). The approach was originally developed for tension headache but has also been used for migraine.

Two studies have shown that cognitive coping training leads to greater improvement in headaches of various types than does a waiting-list control condition. One of the studies used the stress-coping skills variation (Holroyd et al., 1977) while the other used the headache-coping skills variation (Newton & Barbaree, 1987). Comparisons with attention–placebo control procedures have not been forthcoming, but a number of studies have compared cognitive coping training with other treatment techniques that have been shown to be superior to placebo. These studies have been reviewed in previous sections of this chapter and include the finding that this approach is superior to forehead EMG biofeedback training in the treatment of tension headache (Holroyd et al., 1977) and equal in the treatment of migraine to BVP biofeedback training (Knapp & Florin, 1981) and relaxation training (Sorbi & Tellegen, 1986). The findings of Blanchard, Appelbaum, Radnitz, Michultka et al. (1990) suggested that adding cognitive coping training to relaxation training increased its efficacy in the treatment of tension headaches.

The results of this rather limited number of controlled studies have been supplemented by a number of papers reporting case studies or single group outcome studies that suggest that cognitive coping training is an effective treatment for both tension headaches and migraines. Bakal et al. (1981) reported the results of treating a large mixed sample of tension headache, migraine, and combined headache patients with cognitive coping training. Analysis showed significant pre- to posttreatment improvement in headache activity and the gains were maintained at 6-month follow-up. A series of case studies conducted by Anderson, Lawrence, and Olson (1981) showed that both cognitive coping training and relaxation training used alone were effective in reducing head pain, and it seemed that in some instances the combined effects of both treatments facilitated this reduction. Kremsdorf, Kochanowicz, and Costell (1981) reported two tension headache cases treated by forehead EMG biofeedback training and cognitive coping training using a within-series single-case experimental design. The data indicated that headache improvement was associated with the cognitive treatment rather than the biofeedback training.

The review by Blanchard (1987) concluded that relief from tension headaches by cognitive coping training was maintained at 2-year follow-up. Sorbi et al. (1989) reported good maintenance with this approach applied to migraine at 3-year follow-up.

Little evidence is available with respect to the mechanism of cognitive coping training. Newton and Barbaree (1987) assessed cognitive changes associated with cognitive coping training and found that in comparison with untreated controls, treated subjects appraised headache attacks in a more positive manner and reported more frequent occurrence of coping thoughts of a problem-solving nature. Changes in cognitive appraisal were correlated with reduction in headache intensity.

Other Forms of Psychological Treatment

Two other types of biofeedback training have been used in the treatment of headaches. EEG biofeedback has been provided with the goal of alpha enhancement and hence relaxation. Andreychuk and Skriver (1975) found this approach to be as effective for reducing headaches in a sample of migraineurs as thermal biofeedback training and training in self-hypnosis. Cohen et al. (1980), also working with migraine sufferers, showed that EEG biofeedback training was equal to forehead EMG biofeedback training, thermal biofeedback training (differential finger–forehead temperature), and BVP biofeedback training in terms of treatment effectiveness.

Reading (1984) has provided migraineurs with skin conductance biofeedback training. Skin conductance is a measure of sympathetic nervous system activity, so this approach can also be viewed as a form of relaxation training. Reading found skin conductance biofeedback training to be as effective for reducing headaches as forehead EMG biofeedback training and thermal biofeedback training, although none of these three conditions was significantly superior to a false EMG biofeedback condition in this study.

Hypnosis has been used in the treatment of migraine and tension headache. Procedures vary from study to study but usually include training in autohypnosis and suggestions under hypnosis relating to relaxation and use of visual imagery to control headache mechanisms. Three studies have investigated hypnotherapy for migraine. Andreychuk and Skriver (1975) demonstrated that training in self-hypnosis was as effective as thermal biofeedback training and EEG biofeedback training. Anderson, Basker, and Dalton (1975) compared hypnotherapy with administration of a prophylactic medication, namely, prochlorperazine (Stemetil). Hypnotherapy was significantly more effective in reducing the number of attacks. Davidson (1987) reported on a clinical series of migraineurs treated with hypnosis with very positive results. Schlutter et al. (1980) administered hypnotic analgesia, forehead EMG biofeedback training, and forehead EMG biofeedback training, in combination with relaxation training, to a sample of tension headache patients. No significant differences were found between treatments on a variety of pain measures.

Transcendental meditation (TM) is taught according to an internationally standardized procedure by formally trained teachers and is basically made up of exhortations to sit quietly for 20 minutes twice a day using a mantra chosen by the teacher for the meditator. The practice of TM leads to generalized decreased sympathetic nervous system activity (Benson, Malvea, & Graham, 1973). Winkler (1979) treated tension headache patients with TM, forehead EMG biofeedback training, or a control procedure (subjects asked to sit quietly twice a day). In the short term, the two treatment conditions were equally effective and superior to the control condition. At 3- and 7-month follow-ups, differences between the three conditions were no longer present but all had improved. Benson, Klemchuk, and Graham (1974) administered TM to a series of migraineurs with disappointing results, as only 6 out of 17 patients showed clinical improvement.

Mitchell and colleagues have investigated the effects of various behavior therapy strategies on migraine. Mitchell and Mitchell (1971) compared "combined desensitization" (applied relaxation, assertive training, and systematic desensitization) with applied relaxation alone and a no-treatment condition. Combined desensitization differed significantly from the control procedure in terms of decreased frequency and duration of headaches, but relaxation on its own did not. In a further study reported in the same paper, a group receiving combined desensitization did better than groups receiving systematic desensitization or no treatment. Mitchell and White (1977) demonstrated that self-recording and self-monitoring did not affect the frequency of migraine headaches, but training in three behavioral self-management skills led to a 45% reduction in headaches, and training in a further 13 skills led to a 73% reduction.

Turkat and Adams (1982) treated tension headache sufferers with a covert positive reinforcement procedure. "With this technique, the individual imagines performing the target behavior (e.g., pain insensitivity) and then reinforces this behavior by imagining a pleasant image" (p. 191). The results of the study indicated that this procedure was not effective in reducing headaches.

Operant approaches have been used extensively in the treatment of low back pain and two case studies have described successful applications to headaches (Yen & McIntire, 1971; Ramsden et al., 1983). These case studies were reviewed in Chapter 4.

Treatment in Group, Couple, or Family Format

By far the majority of studies on psychological treatment of headaches have used an individual format, but a few studies have evaluated treatment administered to small groups of headache sufferers. The modal number of patients per group across studies is five, although groups with as many as seven to eight patients have been reported. Not surprisingly, group approaches have not employed biofeedback training but have used relaxation training, cognitive coping training, or some combination of two or more techniques.

Williamson et al. (1984) compared two group relaxation programs and a waiting-list control condition using a mixed headache sample. One treatment program was called a self-help condition (4 hours of group meetings encouraging patients to use a self-help manual or relaxation) and the other a therapist-administered condition (12 hours of relaxation training with instructions to practice at home). Results indicated that both treatment conditions were superior to the control condition at 1-month follow-up with the therapist-assisted condition associated with greater treatment gains than the self-helf condition. Janssen and Neutgens (1986) compared autogenic training and progressive relaxation training each administered in a group format. The two types of relaxation training were equally effective for migraine, but progressive relaxation training was more successful in the treatment of tension headache. Murphy, Lehrer, and Jurish (1990) treated tension headache sufferers with either group progressive relaxation training or group cognitive coping training modeled on Holroyd's approach. The proportion of clinically significantly improved patients was greater for the cognitive than for the relaxation condition, and patients in the latter condition only improved within the range commonly observed for medication placebos in previous studies.

Holroyd and Andrasik (1978) reported that adding relaxation training to cognitive coping training in a group format did not lead to greater reduction in tension headaches than did cognitive coping training alone. Relaxation training has been an element of a number of successful group treatment packages which are discussed below (Figueroa, 1982; Martin, Nathan, Milech, & van Keppel, 1989).

The first study to evaluate cognitive coping training administered to small groups was the one just mentioned by Holroyd and Andrasik (1978). This study compared two cognitive coping training conditions (i.e., with or without relaxation training), a headache discussion condition, and a self-monitoring control condition. Both the cognitive conditions and the headache discussion procedure produced substantial reductions in tension headaches that were maintained at a 6-month follow-up, whereas the self-monitoring group showed no change. The results in the former three groups were comparable to results obtained with individual treatment in previous studies by these authors.

Johnson and Thorn (1989) specifically compared cognitive coping training administered individually or in a group format and included a no-treatment control condition. The study provided tentative support that cognitive coping training was effective in reducing headaches, and there was no evidence of differential efficacy between the individual and group formats. As noted above, Murphy et al. (1990) compared group cognitive coping training with group relaxation training and found the former to have an advantage.

Figueroa (1982) constructed a behavioral package consisting of problem-solving techniques, relaxation training, anxiety management, stress inoculation, and pain management techniques with traditional psychotherapy and self-monitoring, the two treatment conditions being administered in a group format. Significant improvement occurred across all headache measures for the behavioral group but not for the other two groups. In a study investigating the relationship between headaches and depression, Martin et al. (1989) compared a treatment approach designed for headaches ("self-management training" consisting of self-monitoring, relaxation training, cognitive restructuring, attention-diversion training, imagery training, and thought management) (Winkler, Underwood, James, & Fatovich, 1982) with a treatment approach designed for depression ("cognitive therapy" consisting of self-monitoring, graded task assignment, activity scheduling, scheduling pleasurable activities, mastery and pleasure technique, identifying automatic thoughts, evaluating thought content, prospective hypothesis testing, and identifying underlying assumptions) (Beck et al., 1979). It should be noted that cognitive therapy as administered in this study was quite different from the techniques collectively referred to as cognitive coping training in this chapter, although there was some overlap. Analysis showed that the two treatments were associated with significant and equal reductions in headache activity, improvement that increased throughout the 12-month follow-up period.

No long-term follow-up studies of group treatment have been reported. Also, the mechanisms of change are unclear. Group relaxation training appears superior to no treatment, but there is no evidence to suggest that it is more than an attention–placebo effect. Although the appropriate controlled comparisons are largely lacking, cognitive coping training administered in a group format does seem to be more than an attention–placebo effect. On the other hand, this form of treatment proved to be no more effective than a headache discussion condition that focused on discussion of the historical roots of symptoms rather than on the development of specific coping skills (Holroyd & Andrasik, 1978). Also, Murphy et al. (1990) reported that cognitive coping training did not appear to produce greater increases in cognitive coping strategies in their study than did relaxation training. Holroyd and Andrasik (1978) did note that all but one participant in their headache discussion condition reported devising cognitive self-control procedures for coping even without training. These authors suggest that their various treatment conditions yielded similar outcomes because of common elements such as the provision of a causal explanation for distressing symptoms that may have served to increase clients' belief in their ability to cope with their symptoms. In turn, these cognitive changes might be expected to lead to a greater initiation and persistence of coping behavior.

Little attention has been given to other formats, but partners or families have been directly involved in the treatment program in some studies. Based on the suppositions that family factors may be implicated in the development of headaches and that headaches impact on the family, couple or family therapy has been recommended by a number of authors. Case studies using this approach have reported mixed results (Roy, 1986, 1989; Simone & Long, 1985). Kunzer (1987) has recommended offering adjuvant marital therapy with biofeedback training to headache sufferers experiencing marital problems in order to reduce posttreatment recidivism.

In view of the trend toward partner involvement in treatment for a variety of conditions (e.g., problem drinking, smoking, obesity, agoraphobia), we tried adding partner involvement to the self-management approach (Martin et al., 1989) discussed above. Partner involvement was instituted in an attempt to increase compliance with treatment demands (e.g., facilitate home relaxation practice). Self-management training accompanied and unaccompanied by partner involvement was compared with a no-treatment control condition, and results indicated that incorporating partner involvement seemed to spoil rather than enhance a successful treatment approach (Kneebone & Martin, 1992). Reasons for this unexpected result are not clear, but we speculated that "dissemination of responsibility" may have been a factor. That is, in the partner-involvement condition, headache sufferers tended to assign responsibility for change to their partners, consequently limiting necessary changes in self-efficacy and locus of control in relation to headaches.

Home-Based Treatment

Pressures for cost containment in health care delivery have encouraged researchers to develop largely home-based minimal-therapist-contact treatments, which are less expensive than clinic-based treatment programs. The first published study reporting on a home-based approach compared clinic-based EMG biofeedback training and stress management training with a home relaxation program for tension headache (Steger & Harper 1980). Only the clinic-based program was successful in significantly reducing headaches, but the authors were sufficiently impressed with the results of their home-based program to suggest that such a program might be a useful starting point, with clinic-based treatment reserved for those who need it.

In another early study, Sherman (1982) provided tension headache sufferers with relaxation tapes and instructions to practice twice daily. All but one subject showed a substantial decrease in headache activity at 6-month follow-up. Kohlenberg and Cahn (1981) contrasted the impact of providing migraineurs with an experimental or control book. The experimental book contained instructions for thermal biofeedback training (with accompanying feedback device), relaxation, and cognitive coping training, while the control book discussed headaches without instructions in behavioral self-help strategies. The authors reported a 62% decrease in headache frequency at 6-month follow-up for subjects using the treatment book compared to a 14% drop for those using the control book.

Since these early studies, a number of reports have appeared in the literature largely from two groups, Blanchard and his colleagues at State University of New York at Albany and Holroyd and his colleagues at Ohio University. The home-based programs have included the following: (1) relaxation training alone (tension headache), (2) cognitive coping training alone (tension headache), (3) relaxation training plus cognitive coping training (tension headache and migraine), (4) relaxation training plus thermal biofeedback training (migraine and combined headache), and (5) relaxation training plus thermal biofeedback training plus cognitive coping training (migraine and combined headache). Home-based programs usually involve approximately three clinic visits supplemented by two or more phone calls and postal exchanges. Patients are typically provided with manuals or workbooks, audiocassette tapes, and feedback devices for programs involving biofeedback training.

Two studies have compared relaxation training delivered in a clinic-based or home-based format to tension headache sufferers (Blanchard, Andrasik, Appelbaum et al., 1985; Teders et al., 1984). Both studies found the home-based approach to be highly effective and virtually equal in reducing headaches to the clinic-based approach, with the home-based approach more cost-effective. Attanasio, Andrasik, and Blanchard (1987) contrasted home-based relaxation training with home-based cognitive coping training and clinic-based relaxation plus cognitive coping training for tension headaches. Patients in all three conditions exhibited significant decreases in headache activity with no significant differences between the groups, although there appeared to be a slight advantage for the cognitive groups and for groups with increased therapist contact. Tobin, Holroyd, Baker, Reynolds, and Holm (1988) compared relaxation training alone with relaxation training plus cognitive coping training, each administered in a home-based format to tension headache sufferers, and found that both treatments yielded substantial reductions in headache activity but patients in the combined treatment recorded significantly larger reductions. On the other hand, Appelbaum et al. (1990) found that adding cognitive coping training to home-based relaxation training conveyed no significant advantage, although both treatment conditions were significantly superior to a headache-monitoring control condition.

The only study evaluating home-based cognitive coping training alone was the one already discussed by Attanasio et al. (1987).

With respect to the combination of home-based relaxation training plus cognitive coping training, one study that has evaluated this combination was discussed above (Tobin et al., 1988). Richardson and McGrath (1989) compared this combination administered with a clinic-based or home-based format and a waiting-list control condition using a sample of migraineurs. Analysis showed that there was a significant reduction in headache activity for both the treatment groups but not for the control group and that treatment for the home-based group was significantly more cost-effective. Holroyd, Nash, Pingel, Cordingley, and Jerome (1991) contrasted home-based relaxation training and cognitive coping training with prophylactic medication (amitriptyline HC1) for tension headache sufferers. Both treatments yielded clinically significant improvements in headache activity, but on measures where differences in treatment effectiveness were observed, the differences favored the psychological approach.

Two studies have compared the combination of relaxation training and thermal biofeedback training administered in a clinic-based or home-based format to migraine and combined headache patients (Blanchard, Andrasik, Appelbaum, et al., 1985; Jurish et al., 1983). Both studies reported the two formats to be equally effective in reducing headaches, with the home-based format more cost-effective. Blanchard et al. (1988) completed a long-term follow-up study and found that the combination of relaxation training and thermal biofeedback training was associated with good maintenance at 2 years for both the clinic-based and the home-based approaches. Holroyd et al. (1988), using a sample of migraine and combined headache patients, compared relaxation and thermal biofeedback training with abortive medication (ergotamine tartrate) accompanied by a compliance-training intervention. The two treatments yielded similar reductions in headache activity.

Blanchard, Appelbaum, Nicholson et al. (1990) evaluated the effect of adding cognitive coping training to the combination of home-based relaxation training and thermal biofeedback training by comparing this combination with and without a cognitive component to a self-monitoring control condition, in a sample of migraine and combined headache patients. The treated groups showed greater reduction in headache activity than did the control group, with no significant difference between the treated groups. Penzien, Johnson, Carpenter, and Holroyd (1990) compared the home-based package of relaxation training, thermal biofeedback training, and cognitive coping training with long-acting propranolol (Inderal) as treatments for migraine. Both treatments were associated with significant reductions in headaches. The two treatments did not differ on most measures of headache activity but propranolol was superior with respect to decrease in weekly peak headaches.

Effects of Treatment on Variables Other than Headaches

A paper by Szajnberg and Diamond (1980) raised the issue of symptom substitution with biofeedback training for headache. These authors interviewed a few individuals who had successfully completed biofeedback training for migraine and reported that 67% experienced some form of "symptom substitution," primarily psychosomatic symptoms or depression, accompanying or following the reduction of headache activity. This paper was criticized on methodological grounds by Haynes and Cuevas (1980), and other studies that have looked for symptom substitution have failed to find support for it (Budzynski et al., 1973). In fact, there is much evidence to suggest that contrary to the findings of Szajnberg and Diamond, psychological treatment for headaches seems to be associated with a reduction in psychosomatic symptoms generally and many beneficial behavioral, affective, and cognitive changes in addition to headache reduction.

Several studies have shown that psychological treaments for headaches lead to decreases in psychosomatic symptoms. Cox et al. (1975) developed a Psychosomatic Checklist consisting of 18 common psychosomatic complaints and showed that scores on this scale were significantly reduced in the treatment of headaches by both EMG biofeedback training and relaxation training. This finding has been replicated with other forms of treatment (e.g., Knapp & Florin, 1981) and alternative measures of psychosomatic symptoms (e.g., Holroyd et al., 1988), although Blanchard, Andrasik et al. (1986) presented data suggesting that the finding may be a measurement artifact.

Most treatment studies require subjects to record medication consumption as well as headaches, and decreased usage of medication following treatment has been reported in investigations of all the major treatment approaches, including EMG biofeedback training (e.g., Budzynski et al.,

1973), thermal biofeedback training (e.g., Gauthier et al., 1981), BVP biofeedback training (e.g., Gauthier et al., 1985), relaxation training (e.g., Cox et al., 1975), cognitive coping training (e.g., Sorbi & Tellegen, 1986), treatment in a group format (e.g., Figueroa, 1982; Holroyd & Andrasik, 1978), and home-based treatment (e.g., Blanchard, Appelbaum, Nicholson et al., 1990; Teders et al., 1984). These data have usually been presented as supporting the efficacy of the treatment approaches, although given the evidence reviewed in Chapter 4 that excessive consumption of certain drugs can induce headaches, such an interpretation must be viewed with some caution.

Radnitz, Appelbaum, Blanchard, Elliott, and Andrasik (1988) assessed the effects of psychological treatment on four types of pain behavior: medication consumption, avoidance behavior, verbal complaint behavior, and nonverbal complaint behavior. Significant reductions occurred following treatment on all four types of behavior even though these behaviors were not targeted. Also, significant correlations were found between headache percentage improvement scores and improvement scores for each of the four types of pain behavior. Philips (1987b) also reported a reduction in avoidance behavior associated with behavioral treatment in a mixed pain sample that included headache sufferers. Sorbi and Tellegen (1986) focused on social behavior and found that patients receiving relaxation training became more socially withdrawn but patients who underwent cognitive coping training increased their social assertiveness.

With respect to changes in mood and emotional symptoms, a number of studies have demonstrated that psychological treatment for headaches is associated with decreases in depression (e.g., Martin et al., 1989; Cox & Thomas, 1981; Sovak, Kunzel, Sternbach, & Dalessio, 1981). Other studies have shown reductions in anxiety (e.g., Blanchard, Andrasik, et al., 1986; Knapp & Florin, 1981). Positive changes have also been reported in terms of fatigue and irritability (Knapp & Florin, 1981; Knapp 1982) and anger (Holroyd et al., 1991). Published correlations between changes in headaches and changes in mood have failed to achieve significance (e.g., Cox & Thomas, 1981; Martin et al., 1989; Blanchard, Steffek, Jaccard, & Nicholson, 1991).

With respect to cognitive changes associated with the psychological treatment of headaches, studies have demonstrated that subjects shift toward a more internal locus of control as measured by general scales (Cox et al., 1975), health scales (Mizener et al., 1988), and headache scales (Penzien et al., 1990). Treatment leads to enhanced self-efficacy to cope with headaches (Holroyd et al., 1984), greater perceived control over pain (Philips, 1987b), and increased ability to cope with headaches (Murphy et al., 1990). Significant correlations have been reported between changes in headaches and these cognitive changes (Holroyd et al., 1984; Mizener et al., 1988).

Evidence is also available to suggest that psychological treatment can alter cognitive reactions to stressors. Newton and Barbaree (1987) reported that cognitive coping training led to a mixed sample of headache sufferers appraising headache attacks in a more positive manner and having a more frequent occurrence of coping thoughts of a problem-solving nature. Changes in cognitive appraisal were correlated with reductions in headache intensity following treatment. Mizener et al. (1988) found a trend for migraineurs treated by thermal biofeedback training to increase the use of coping self-statements and to decrease catastrophizing. Sorbi et al. (1989) reported that migraineurs treated with cognitive coping training improved in terms of assertiveness and active problem solving.

A few studies have suggested that psychological treatment for headaches is associated with changes in personality. Budzynski et al. (1973) and Grazzi, Frediani, Zappacosta, Boiardi, and Bussone (1988) reported that EMG biofeedback training resulted in a significant decrease in hysteria; Janssen (1983) reported that combined forehead EMG biofeedback training and relaxation training resulted in decreases in neuroticism and somatization. Sovak et al. (1981) found that migraineurs who responded to biofeedback training improved in terms of neuroticism. Knapp and Florin (1981) reported that cognitive coping training led to increased positive self-evaluation.

Predictors of Change and Client–Treatment Matching

The most comprehensive study of outcome prediction was carried out by Blanchard, Andrasik, Arena et al. (1983). These authors used canonical discriminant-function analysis to predict the response of a mixed sample of headache patients to biofeedback training and relaxation training. Pretreatment measures were classified into four sets. Headache history variables correctly classified as improved or unimproved 87.5% to 95.2% of cases. Data from baseline headache diaries correctly classified 66.7% to 70.3% of tension headache cases but failed to classify migraineurs at beyond chance level. Scores on six psychological tests resulted in 75.7% to 90.6% correct classification, and psychophysiological measures predicted outcome correctly for 76.2% to 89.7% of cases.

The approach used by Blanchard and his colleagues is statistically sophisticated but lacking in clinical utility as it requires complex calculations to classify a patient. Much data exists, however, on individual predictors that are more useful.

In the meta-analytic review of EMG biofeedback training and relaxation training for tension headache sufferers by Holroyd and Penzien (1986), studies using younger samples gained superior results. A number of studies have reported age to be a significant predictor of treatment success (e.g., Blanchard, Andrasik, Evans, Neff et al., 1985; Diamond, Medina, Diamond-Falk, & DeVeno, 1979), but other studies have found nonsignificant relationships (e.g., Martin et al., 1989). Blanchard, Andrasik, Evans, and Hillhouse (1985) completed a retrospective review of 11 older (60 years or greater) headache patients treated by a combination of biofeedback and relaxation training and found that only 18.2% were clinically improved after treatment. On the other hand, a series of recent prospective studies with the elderly have reported clinical improvement rates varying between 50% and 70% (Arena, Hightower, & Chong, 1988; Arena, Hannah, Bruno, & Meador, 1991; Kabela, Blanchard, Appelbaum, & Nicholson, 1989).

The review by Holroyd and Penzien (1986) also found sex to be an outcome predictor (superior response for females), although the relationship between sex and improvement ($r = -.24$) was smaller than the relationship between age and improvement ($r = -.55$). Women were found to improve more than men in response to biofeedback training in a study by Diamond et al. (1979).

Most researchers have administered different treatments to different diagnostic groups (tension vs. migraine and combined headaches), but when researchers have given the same treatment to different diagnostic groups they have usually found no evidence of differential efficacy. Bakal and colleagues found no difference in outcome between diagnostic groups in response to EMG biofeedback training (Bakal & Kaganov, 1977) or cognitive coping training (Bakal et al., 1981). I obtained similar null findings in response to self-management training and cognitive therapy (Martin et al., 1989). Williamson et al. (1984) reported that headache diagnosis did not predict response to their group relaxation program.

Janssen and Neutgens (1986) did not focus on the differential response of diagnostic groups to treatment procedures, but their data seemed to show that no differential response occurred for progressive relaxation training but a differential response occurred for autogenic training with tension headache sufferers responding less well than migraineurs or combined headache patients. The total ineffectiveness of autogenic training as a treatment for tension headaches was a surprising finding in view of earlier research indicating that this approach was effective (e.g., Haynes et al., 1975). Gauthier, Fradet, and Roberge (1988) reported that patients diagnosed as "classical migraine" improved significantly more with thermal or BVP biofeedback training than did patients diagnosed as "common migraine."

Two studies have suggested that biofeedback training and relaxation training are less effective when headaches are associated with menstruation (Solbach, Sargent, & Coyne, 1984; Szekeley et al., 1986). Two recent studies have tested this possibility more rigorously, however, and have shown that psychological treatment is as effective in reducing menstrual migraine as it is in reducing nonmenstrual migraine (Gauthier, Fournier, & Roberge, 1991; Kim & Blanchard, 1992).

In one of my studies, we investigated the prognostic significance of the antecedent and consequences dimensions that emerged from factor analysis of functional characteristics (Martin, Milech, & Nathan, 1992). Scores on the antecedent dimension Negative Affect correlated significantly with reduction in headache frequency ($r = .31$), and scores on the consequences dimension Encourage Rest correlated with two indices of headache improvement, namely, reduction in average pain ($r = .32$) and reduction in duration of pain ($r = .34$). Hence, headaches that were precipitated by negative emotions and headaches that were followed by the supportive partner's reaction of encouraging the sufferers to stop what they were doing and sit or lie down responded best to psychological treatments. Although these correlations are not high, they are higher than correlations obtained between headache improvement on the one hand and diagnosis, age, and chronicity on the other (Martin et al., 1989).

One of the more solid findings with respect to prediction of outcome is that individuals who experience continuous or near continuous headaches respond less well to psychological treatments than do individuals who suffer from episodic headaches. This relationship has been demonstrated for biofeedback and relaxation training (Blanchard, Appelbaum, Radnitz, Jaccard, & Dentinger, 1989), cognitive coping training (Bakal et al., 1981), and home-based treatment (Holroyd et al., 1988). In a similar vein, levels of pretreatment headache activity have emerged as a predictor in some studies, with high levels associated with poor response (Jacob, Turner, Szekely, & Eidelman, 1983; Tobin et al., 1988). Also, high levels of medication consumption have been shown to predict poor response to biofeedback and relaxation training (Diamond et al., 1979; Michultka, Blanchard, Appelbaum, Jaccard, & Dentinger, 1989).

Numerous studies have reported that the presence of depressive symptoms prior to treatment suggests poor prognosis (e.g., Jacob et al., 1983; Levine, 1984; Blanchard, Andrasik, Neff, Teders et al., 1982). Blanchard, Andrasik, Evans, Neff et al. (1985) found that high scores in terms of trait anxiety, hypochondriasis, and hysteria were associated with less improvement than were low scores on these personality variables. A study by Gatchel, Deckel, Weinberg, and Smith (1985) demonstrated that a number of scales on the Millon Behavioral Health Inventory significantly predicted response to treatment, in particular, the Emotional Vulnerability scale.

Two patient variables that have been reported as unrelated to treatment outcome are treatment credibility (Gauthier et al., 1985) and therapeutic expectancies (Murphy et al., 1990).

A number of studies have investigated therapist effects with mixed results. Andrasik and Holroyd (1980a) and Gauthier et al. (1981) reported no significant therapist effects, but Holroyd and Andrasik (1978) found that one therapist obtained somewhat larger reductions in headache activity than did the other therapist, and Martin et al. (1989) found significant therapist effects on some outcome measures but not on others. Unfortunately, it is quite unclear why the patients of some therapists may improve more than the patients of others. Blanchard, Andrasik, Neff et al. (1983) found no relationship between the therapist variables of level of experience, warmth, competence, and helpfulness as perceived by the patient and response to biofeedback and relaxation training. Similar null findings were reported by Holroyd and Andrasik (1978) for warmth, empathy, and skilfulness and by Martin et al. (1989) for warmth, empathy, genuineness, competence, persuasiveness, confidence, likability, supportiveness, sensitivity, and understandability.

With respect to treatment variables, the review of Holroyd and Penzien (1986) reported that across studies, treatment outcome was not related to type of intervention, length of treatment, or whether efforts were made to facilitate transfer of training. Several investigators have found regularity of home relaxation practice to be a significant predictor of treatment success (e.g., Blanchard, Andrasik, Neff et al., 1983; Reinking & Hutchings, 1981). On the other hand, a recent study by Solbach, Sargent, and Coyne (1989) reported that quality of home practice, as measured by variables such as changes in feelings associated with practice, was more important than quantity of home practice. Blanchard, Nicholson et al. (1991) compared progressive relaxation training administered with or without home practice and found no significant difference in terms of headache reduction between the two conditions, although there was a trend favoring home practice.

As the literature on predictors of response to various treatments develops, one obvious offshoot is client–treatment matching strategies that link clients to the treatment approach most likely to benefit them. One example is provided by my study comparing self-management training with cognitive therapy (Martin et al., 1989). In this study, pretreatment depression was a significant predictor of response to self-management training replicating a common finding, but pretreatment depression was not a significant predictor of response to cognitive therapy. Conversely, chronicity was a significant predictor for cognitive therapy (high chronicity, more improvement) but not for self-management training. These findings raise the possibility that self-management training or some other standard behavioral technique such as biofeedback training or relaxation training may be appropriate for nondepressed headache sufferers, but cognitive therapy may be the treatment of choice for more chronic headache patients with depressive symptoms (perhaps one third to one half of chronic headache sufferers).

Another example arose from the study by Tobin et al. (1988). These authors found that high pretreatment levels of headache activity and daily life stress were associated with a poor response to relaxation training but were unrelated to patient's response to combined relaxation training plus cognitive coping training, suggesting that the combined treatment was preferable for patients with elevated headache activity and stress. A parallel finding was reported by Sorbi et al. (1989) in that relaxation training worked best for headache sufferers experiencing little external stress, whereas self-motivation was the best predictor of response to cognitive coping training (high motivation was associated with success).

Summary

There is now strong evidence available that several psychological treatment approaches are effective in reducing headaches (tension and migraine), and that these gains are at least maintained for 12 months. The beneficial effects achieved with these treatments are more than attention–placebo effects. Most of the research has concentrated on the individually administered treatment approaches of biofeedback training, relaxation training, and cognitive coping training, but there is also support for treatment administered in a group format and home-based approaches. Meta-analytic reviews have calculated average percentage of improvement rates across studies, associated with biofeedback training and relaxation training, varying between 45% and 65%, in contrast to rates associated with placebo procedures varying between 12% and 38%. It should be noted, however, that these averages have been obtained from studies with varied improvement rates, (e.g., the range of such scores for active treatment was from 13% to 94% in the review by Holroyd and Penzien [1986])

In addition to reducing headache activity, psychological treatments lead to many other positive changes. Treatment is associated with decreased consumption of medication and changes in pain behaviors such as avoidance behavior and verbal and nonverbal complaint behavior. Treatment is also associated with decreases in negative moods such as depression and anxiety and various cognitive changes. Cognitive changes include a shift toward a more internal locus of control and enhanced self-efficacy to cope with headaches. Also, treatment is associated with alterations in cognitive reactions to stress, such as changes in appraisal and coping processes. Reduced neuroticism, hysteria, somatization, and psychosomatic symptoms have been reported in treatment studies.

There is evidence to suggest that the treatment gains associated with thermal biofeedback training, BVP biofeedback training, relaxation training, and cognitive coping training are maintained for at least 3 to 6 years.

Improvement achieved via EMG biofeedback training seems to progressively deteriorate after 12 months, although not back to pretreatment levels.

Comparisons between different forms of treatment have rarely produced differential effects. A few studies have found one treament superior to another, but this has usually resulted from one treatment's uncharacteristically poor results. On the other hand, many studies have used small subject samples and therefore have lacked the statistical power necessary to demonstrate significant differences. Treatments vary with respect to the quantity and quality of evidence testifying to their efficacy. Those in the section "Other Forms of Psychological Treatment" have less support. As noted above, a review of the long-term effects of psychological treatment suggests that improvement achieved with EMG biofeedback training may not last as long as improvement achieved by other forms of treatment.

Although most treatments seem equally effective in terms of ability to reduce headaches, they differ in other respects. Contrast, for example, relaxation training, which requires no equipment and relatively little expertise to administer, with BVP biofeedback training, which requires complex equipment and considerable technical skills to carry out. Group treatment seems a more efficient format than individual treatment if there are large numbers of headache patients seeking help, and home-based approaches are more cost-effective than clinic-based approaches.

It is quite unclear how psychological treatments achieve their effects or even whether the different treatments operate via the same or different mechanisms. The evidence seems to refute the rationale of EMG biofeedback training that improvement in headaches is achieved by learning to relax overly tense pericranial muscles. Whether the mechanism of thermal biofeedback or BVP biofeedback training involves learned control of some cardiovascular process is not known because the evidence is mixed and incomplete. The problems discussed in Chapter 3 concerning difficulties in measuring the state of dilation of arteries and variations in vascular models of headaches all render investigation of vascular treatment mechanisms difficult.

Many researchers have responded to the negative findings with respect to the association between headache change and physiological change by proposing that headache improvement is mediated by cognitive mechanisms such as changes in locus of control and feelings of self-efficacy. This approach seems highly plausible and correlative evidence exists that supports the importance of cognitive change. The data are far from complete, however.

Studies of predictors of treatment response have shown that poor outcome is associated with continuous headaches, high medication consumption, high pretreatment headache activity, and high pretreatment depression. The literature suggests that young patients fare better than older patients, and the response of females is superior to that of males. Quantity or quality of home relaxation practice is associated with outcome. Variables that seem unrelated to treatment response include diagnosis, patients' expectations, and therapist variables such as warmth, empathy, and competence.

Early findings on client–treatment matching suggest the value of cognitive approaches for more complicated cases. For example, cognitive therapy may be the treatment of choice for more chronic, depressed headache sufferers, and adding cognitive coping training to relaxation training seems desirable for patients with high pretreatment headache activity and daily life stress.

II

PSYCHOLOGICAL ASSESSMENT OF HEADACHES

Lord how my head aches!
What a head have I!
It beats as it would fall
in twenty pieces.
    —WILLIAM SHAKESPEARE

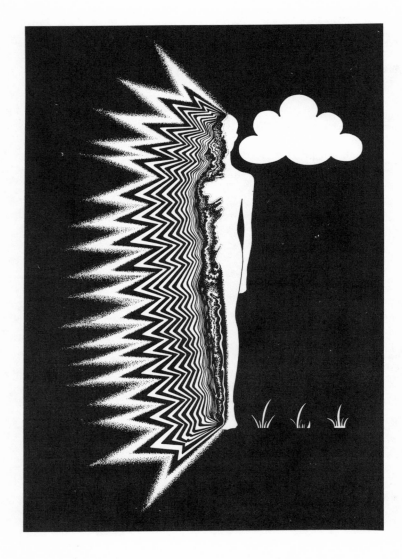

6

Preliminary Considerations and General Assessment Methods

Part II discusses how to complete a psychological assessment of headaches from a functional perspective and provides two case examples of the approach. How to use this information to design an appropriate treatment program is described at the beginning of Part III.

The two main techniques used in the functional assessment of headaches are interviewing and self-monitoring, and they are discussed in this chapter. There are many other, more specialized techniques that can be used to advantage at least with some headache sufferers and they are discussed in the next chapter.

Given the large amount of information needed from an interview and the necessity for clients to engage in self-monitoring to complete a functional analysis, this approach requires a minimum of two assessment sessions. A third session is often needed when headache problems are more complex (e.g., two distinct types of headaches) or patients are less adept at answering questions.

A number of factors need consideration before carrying out a functional analysis, or at least at an early stage of the assessment, so these are discussed prior to focusing on interviewing and self-monitoring.

Preliminary Considerations

Collaboration with Medical Practitioners

Headaches may result from a large number of organic disorders and diseases, including head trauma, vascular disorders (e.g., cerebrovascular disease, hematoma, hemorrhage, thrombosis, aneurysm, arteritis), brain tumor, infections (viral, bacterial, etc.), metabolic disorder, nose and sinus disease, eye and ear disorders, trigeminal neuralgia, and temporomandibular joint disease. Despite the diversity of organic problems that can cause headaches, such headaches are apparently rare. Diamond (1979) has estimated that collectively they account for only 2% of cases seen by family physicians. Presumably they constitute a smaller percentage of cases seen by other types of health professionals. Headaches can also occur as side effects of drugs or from the overuse of, or withdrawal from, medication taken to prevent or abort headaches (see Chapter 4).

The potential for headaches to result from organic factors makes collaboration with medical practitioners a necessity. Certainly it is essential that headache sufferers are seen by a physician prior to psychological treatment. Ideally, headache sufferers should be seen by an appropriate medical specialist (i.e., a neurologist) who will take a detailed history, carry out a general physical and neurological examination, and organize additional investigations as required. The most important of these is cranial computerized axial tomography (CAT) scanning; other investigations such as spinal puncture and cerebral angiography may be necessary in occasional cases.

Blanchard and Andrasik (1985) published a list compiled by a neurologist of signs and symptoms for which nonmedical practitioners should be especially alert. A modified version of this list appears in Table 6.1. It is particularly important to refer headache sufferers to a neurologist in the circumstances described in the table. Headaches that cause the greatest concern are those with a short history of increasing severity.

Low-Cost Approaches to Psychological Management of Headaches

Given that a functional approach to headache management as outlined in this section involves professionals working with patients on an individual basis, using relatively high-level skills, and two or three assessment sessions prior to commencing treatment, it is appropriate to consider less costly psychological management approaches before embarking on a full functional analysis. The literature reviewed in Chapter 5 shows that relaxation training administered in a standardized format is a reasonably effective treatment for headaches, particularly for less severe cases and for headaches unassociated with high levels of daily stress. This approach has the merit of requiring (1) minimal psychological assessment, (2) relatively low levels of professional expertise to administer, and (3) no equipment. On the other hand, it does seem a somewhat superficial approach to be used in isolation as a treatment for headaches given the diverse controlling variables and implications of headaches discussed in Chapter 4.

TABLE 6.1. Signs and Symptoms That Should Prompt Referral to a Neurologist

Onset factors
 1. The headaches are of recent onset (viz. less than 6 months) or have changed significantly within the previous 6 to 12 months.
 2. The headaches began after some trauma to the head, especially if the individual was rendered unconscious.
 3. The headaches had a sudden onset under conditions of exertion such as lifting, during sexual intercourse, or during a heated argument.

Headache symptoms
 4. The headaches are associated with any sensory or motor deficits such as weakness or numbness in an extremity, other than the typical visual prodromata of classic migraine, or aphasia or slurred speech.
 5. The headaches are unilateral and have always been on the same side.
 6. The headaches are constant and unremitting.
 7. The headaches are worse in the morning and become less severe during the day.
 8. The headaches appear to fall into the tension headache category but are accompanied by vomiting.

Patient variables
 9. Headaches occurring in individuals who have previously been treated for any type of cancer.
10. Headaches occurring in association with noticeable changes in personality or behavior or decreased memory or other intellectual functioning.
11. Headaches occurring as a new complaint in individuals over 60 years of age.
12. Headaches occurring in individuals with a family history of cerebral aneurysm, other vascular abnormalities, or polycystic kidneys.

Adapted from Blanchard and Andrasik (1985).

Treatment in a group format is quite effective and is likely to be more cost-effective than treatment administered on an individual basis. Of course this approach is only possible if there are several patients who require treatment for headaches at the same time.

Treatment using a minimal-therapist-contact home-based format is more cost-effective than clinic-based treatment and therefore worth considering. Such an approach requires the use of various materials to guide the patients' efforts outside the clinic (manuals, tapes, etc.) and these are not widely available. Also, minimal-therapist-contact formats are not always acceptable to patients or health professionals.

Of course, the less costly approaches listed above are not necessarily alternatives to a functional approach. One possibility is to use one of them in the first instance, reserving a functional approach for patients who do not respond well to treatment.

Techniques That Can Be Used Prior to First Interview

It is worth considering an information exchange with patients prior to the first interview. Materials can be sent through the mail or given to them in the clinic before the interview. I have prepared an information sheet for patients to read while they are in the waiting room (see Appendix 3). This sheet orients patients to the forthcoming assessment and treatment sessions which is a useful exercise because many patients who see psychologists for headache treatment arrive with either erroneous expectations or no expectations what-soever. Patients can take the sheets home for rereading and to show their partner.

On the assessment side, self-monitoring forms and instructions can be sent through the mail to be completed over 1 or 2 weeks prior to first appointment. This is a dubious strategy, because patients often struggle to understand or fail to appreciate the significance of instructions delivered only in written form, but it can be a viable option if accompanied by a phone call. Questionnaires may be administered prior to the first interview as a screening function (e.g., instruments for assessing depression and anxiety, as mood problems often accompany chronic headaches).

A number of headache clinics have patients complete a computerized questionnaire prior to being examined by a physician. Early examples of such questionnaires required the presence of trained assistants (e.g., Freemon, 1968; Toole, Brady, Cochrane, & Olmos, 1974), but more recent examples eliminate the need for assistants as the computer communicates directly with the patient (e.g., Bana, Leviton, Swidler, Slack, & Graham, 1980; Bana, Leviton, Slack, Geer, & Graham, 1981). Most computer-based approaches aim to provide physicians with headache history information and provisional diagnosis. Published evaluations of this approach report good patient and physician acceptance but rather mixed findings with respect to the utility of the information produced by the current generation of programs (Bana et al., 1980; Bana et al., 1981). One article has described a computerized question-naire that is more oriented toward behavioral assessment than toward di-agnosis, but the program was written for use with school-age children rather than adults (Leviton, Slack, Masek, Bana, & Graham, 1984).

A recent study has promoted a novel approach to collecting information before assessment by a clinician. Bana, Graham, and Spierings (1988) ask their patients simply to write about themselves. These authors argued that "the autobiographies which (the patients) eagerly supplied were amazingly frank and helpful in revealing details of their lives and feelings of a sort considered relevant to the management of the patient with headaches" (p. 403).

Interviewing and Questionnaires

Questionnaires

A number of researchers have published self-administered questionnaires in full or provided enough information on questions and responses to enable readers to reconstruct the questionnaires. These questionnaires include the following: 14 items (Bakal & Kaganov, 1979), 14 items (Attanasio & Andrasik, 1987), 16 items (Peck & Attfield, 1981), 20 items (Blanchard & Andrasik, 1985), 24 items (Thompson & Collins, 1979), and 26 items (Thompson & Figueroa, 1980). The questionnaires typically focus on headache parameters (frequency, intensity, duration) and symptoms and can be completed in a few minutes. Some questionnaires are designed to lead to a diagnosis. Most published reports include percentage of response data and some include additional information such as the test–retest reliability coefficients for each item (Thompson & Collins, 1979; Attanasio & Andrasik, 1987) and correlations between items (Bakal & Kaganov, 1979).

In addition to the self-administered questionnaire listed previously, Blanchard and Andrasik (1985) have published the "headache history" form which they have used in their research program. This instrument needs to be administered in a semistructured interview format and takes 60 to 90 minutes to complete.

Included in Appendix 4 is a revised version of the Psychological Assessment of Headache Questionnaire (PAHQ) that I have used in my research program over the last 8 years (e.g., Martin, Milech, & Nathan, 1992). This questionnaire needs to be administered by an interviewer, although we have developed abbreviated versions that can be self-administered. Questions that provide information with respect to signs and symptoms that prompt referral to a neurologist (see Table 6.1) are denoted by A (Alert), and questions that enable an IHS diagnosis to be made are denoted by D (Diagnosis). The PAHQ is divided into two parts, the first focuses on personal and social history and the second on the headaches. The main aims of part I are to provide a broad psychosocial context for the headache assessment and to begin eliciting information related to danger signs and symptoms.

The second part of the PAHQ begins with the question whether the patient can identify more than one type of headache. This question is important because in our experience, approximately 50% of chronic headache sufferers respond affirmatively and can indeed describe two types of headaches which differ from each other from both a symptomatological and a functional perspective. Both types of headaches need assessment, and this can be achieved by completing part II for each type of headache successively (the method we use) or concurrently.

The second part is divided into three sections: A, headaches and associated symptoms; B, functional analysis; and C, assessment and treatment history. The primary purpose of Section A is to enable a diagnosis to be made on the basis of the criteria listed in the IHS headache classification system. Of the many different types of headaches listed in this system and reproduced in Appendix 1, the categories of most interest to psychologists are all variations of tension-type headaches and some forms of migraine. Cases of migraine without aura are appropriate for referral to psychologists as well as some cases of migraine with aura (e.g., migraine with typical aura, the commonest form of migraine with aura). Other types of migraine with aura are less likely to be referred because they occur less frequently and therefore are not so incapacitating and are more likely to respond to pharmacological prophylactic approaches. Guidelines are provided in Appendix 2 that enable headaches to be diagnosed into the two main types of migraine (migraine without aura and migraine with typical aura) and three types of tension-type headache (episodic tension-type headache, chronic tension-type headache, and headache of the tension-type not fulfilling above criteria) based on the responses to questions in section A. It should be emphasized, however, that in making these diagnoses, the IHS system assumes that other headache types have been eliminated via history taking, general physical and neurological examinations, and appropriate investigations. Hence, these guidelines apply to differentiating between the common types of headaches only after headaches of organic origin have been ruled out.

Section B is the longest section of the PAHQ and is concerned with a functional analysis of the headaches. The major objective of a functional analysis is to understand the variance in the problem behavior. The section begins by asking about patterns in headache activity (are they associated with particular times of day, particular days, periods of the month, seasons of the year). The next set of questions pertains to headaches and sleep. These questions are included to explore the impact of headaches on sleep, whether headache sufferers react to headache-induced sleep problems in optimal ways, and whether partners may be reinforcing headaches associated with waking.

The functional analysis then focuses on changes in headache activity, both headaches beginning or getting worse and headaches diminishing or ending. Factors that precipitate or aggravate headaches are considered, followed by factors that relieve headaches. The next set of questions pertains to the immediate consequences of headache change, again both for headaches beginning or getting worse and for headaches diminishing or ending. The consequences are explored both for the sufferer and for others with whom they interact regularly. The emphasis is on looking for relatively maladaptive reactions as discussed in Chapter 4.

The next set of questions considers the long-term consequences of the headaches for the sufferer and for significant others. The history of the headaches is then pursued and questions are directed at initial onset and at periods in which the headaches changed for better or for worse. The final questions in the functional analysis section ask about relatives and close friends with headaches, as this information is relevant to issues of susceptibility or modeling as a contributory learning process.

Some data from the PAHQ have been published (discussed in Chapter 4). Responses to the questions on factors that precipitate or aggravate headaches and the questions on how sufferers and significant others respond to headaches have been factor-analyzed to reveal patterns of antecedents and consequences (Martin, Milech, & Nathan, 1992).

RELIABILITY AND VALIDITY OF HEADACHE QUESTIONNAIRES

Although self-administered questionnaires are commonly used in headache research, studies assessing their reliability and validity have cast some doubt on the soundness of the data they yield. Thompson and Collins (1979) readministered a headache questionnaire 3 months after first administration and found that test–retest correlations for the 31 responses (some of the 24 items had multiple responses) were all significant at the 1% level and varied from .37 to .90. Andrasik and Holroyd (1980c) assessed test–retest reliability after a 2-week interval and reported correlations of .66, .77, and .84 for questions on headache intensity, duration, and frequency, respectively. These authors also compared subjects in terms of levels across the two occasions, however, and found significant differences in intensity and a trend for differences in frequency and duration. Attanasio and Andrasik (1987) readministered a headache questionnaire at intervals of 1 week, 4 weeks, and 8 weeks. Generally, test–retest reliabilities were high for the 31 responses, but reliability was low for some items, particularly in the symptomatological area such as site of pain and quality of pain.

A recent study by Rasmussen, Jensen, and Olesen (1991) compared diagnosis by self-administered questionnaire with diagnosis by clinical interview according to the IHS classification criteria. These authors concluded that self-administered questionnaires were unsatisfactory tools for diagnosis.

We have assessed the social validity of antecedent data generated from the PAHQ (Watts, 1991). Headache sufferers and their partners completed questions, and responses were compared. Factor scores were calculated for each of the five antecedent dimensions discussed in Chapter 4. Correlations were first calculated between the factor scores of headache sufferers and their partners for each dimension. All correlations were significant at the .001 level and were as follows: Negative Affect, $r = .38$; Visual Disturbance, $r = .45$; Somatic Stress, $r = .43$; Environmental Stress, $r = .44$; and Consumatory Stimuli, $r = .36$. Next, correlations were calculated for each subject across the five dimensions. Seventy-eight percent of subjects had correlations above .40, and the mean correlation was .59 ($p < .01$).

Andrasik and Holroyd (1980c) assessed the concurrent validity of questionnaire data by comparing measures of headache frequency, intensity, and duration derived from responses to questionnaires versus self-monitoring. Two correlations calculated from an outpatient sample were very low (.18 and .09) and nonsignificant, and only two of six correlations calculated from two student samples were significant. Similarly, Attanasio and Andrasik (1987) reported little correspondence between questionnaire estimates of headache parameters and data obtained via self-monitoring.

Of course, discrepancies between questionnaire and self-monitoring data do not necessarily mean that the former are inaccurate. After all, self-monitoring may be associated with problems such as reactivity (i.e., the act of recording changing the variable being recorded). Given that questionnaire responses involve a memory component whereas self-monitoring minimizes the need for recall, it does seem likely that the latter is more accurate. Consequently, the researchers who have investigated the concurrent validity of questionnaire data have recommended that it should be supplemented by self-monitoring data wherever possible. Interestingly, medical researchers investigating the IHS headache classification system have also recommended the use of headache diaries as a method of improving diagnostic reliability (Iversen et al., 1990).

Researchers have assessed the reliability of only a limited number of questionnaire items and evaluated the validity of an even more limited number of items. Clinical experience suggests, however, that the limitations of questionnaire data implied by the research findings may have wide applicability. In my experience, for example, it is common to find that the headache cycles identified by patients in response to questions are not supported by self-monitoring data (e.g., headaches are less closely associated with the menstrual cycle than is commonly reported and differentiation between headache activity on weekdays and weekends is less apparent than often reported). The problem from the clinical perspective is that many questions cannot be easily verified by alternative assessment methods such as self-monitoring.

Interviewing

The distinction between questionnaires and interviews can, of course, become blurred because questionnaires such as Blanchard and Andrasik's headache history and our PAHQ have not been designed for self-administration and amount to semistructured interviews.

When I see patients in a clinical setting I arrange for them to read the Preassessment Patient Information Sheet (see Appendix 3) prior to the interview. Consequently, the interview begins with my asking whether they have any questions arising from the sheet or wish to discuss any of the sheet's content.

I then outline the agenda for the next two sessions, indicating that today's session will begin with a request to briefly describe their headache problem. This will be followed by questions about their background. I explain that this part of the session will not focus on headaches but on obtaining information necessary for the headache assessment. I usually give one or two examples of why it is necessary to collect background information. I explain that the assessment will then proceed to questions about the headaches and this will begin in Session 1 and continue in Session 2. I indicate that patients will need to record their headaches in diaries, and that instructions on how to do this will be given at the end of the first session so that they can start completing the diaries immediately. I also mention that I would like them to complete some questionnaires between Sessions 1 and 2.

Most patients are comfortable with outlining their headache problem, but if they want more guidance I say something like, "I want to hear about what *you* think is important but you might consider describing your headaches, telling me about what you think causes them, and briefly summarizing the history of the problem."

I include this general, open-ended question at the beginning of the assessment for a number of reasons. First, headache sufferers are often able, within the space of a few minutes, to give a very coherent picture of their headaches, including some penetrating insights into mechanisms. This probably occurs because the patients have been rehearsing extensively what they are going to say prior to the interview. A second related reason for asking this question is that the answer helps orient the clinician for the forthcoming assessment and sensitizes him or her to salient issues. Third, patients referred for headaches are usually bursting to talk about their headaches, so they need to get this off their chest before they are asked questions about their personal and social history. Finally, beginning the assessment with this question enables the clinician to focus all his or her attention on the patient without being distracted by note taking, as notes will be recorded when the information is repeated during the subsequent detailed questioning. Because the account offered by patients is often such a good summary of the headache problem, I usually record it on tape.

After the patient has described his or her headache problem, I proceed to complete a personal and social history and headache assessment following the format of the PAHQ. The main problem in following the format is that patients usually answer questions by volunteering too much information, a lot of which pertains to future questions rather than to the one at hand. However, if this tendency is identified early, most patients are able to adjust their responses accordingly.

I discontinue the assessment approximately 15 minutes before the scheduled end of the session to allow for instructions in self-monitoring and completion of questionnaires and for opportunities for patients to ask questions. Most commonly, the session ends at the division between sections A and B of part II of the questionnaire. At this point I initiate completion of the "daily cards," described in the next section. I ask patients to complete the BDI

(Beck, Ward, Mendelsohn, Mock, & Erbaugh, 1961) and the State–Trait Anxiety Inventory (STAI) (Spielberger, Gorsuch, & Lushene, 1970). As depression and anxiety commonly occur in association with chronic headaches, these questionnaires are administered as screening instruments.

Session 2 begins with checking the completed self-monitoring and questionnaires. The aims are to detect and remedy any errors that have occurred and to reinforce patients for complying with instructions. Patients are also given the opportunity to correct or add to information they gave in Session 1. Session 2 then continues the headache assessment.

So far, this section has focused on interviewing the headache sufferer. It was pointed out in a previous section that the answers given to questions on headaches may not be entirely reliable or valid. One approach to this problem is to attempt to corroborate information by interviewing significant others. Questions that seem particularly appropriate for this purpose include those on screening (e.g., changes in personality, behavior, memory, and intellectual functioning) and those in the functional analysis section, with obvious exceptions (e.g., those pertaining to the patients' thoughts and imagery).

There seem to be pros and cons associated with involving partners. Advantages include gaining additional information to aid conceptualizing the problem and eliciting their support for the treatment program. On the other hand, we have found that involving partners in treatment can be detrimental, a finding that we suspect arises from disseminating responsibility for headache improvement from the sufferer to the partner (Kneebone & Martin, 1992).

I discuss the pros and cons with the patient at the end of the first assessment session and indicate my willingness to see the partner—without stressing its importance. The decision is left to the patient and his or her partner.

Self-Monitoring

Perhaps the first point to be made about self-monitoring headache activity is that individuals suffering from headaches seem to have an amazing capacity for keeping records of their headaches. I have conducted several research studies that involved having headache sufferers complete extensive daily self-monitoring tasks including hourly pain ratings over periods of up to 3 months with minimal contact and no treatment. Clinically, it is striking how easy it is to persuade headache sufferers to self-monitor their headaches compared to convincing individuals with other types of problems to carry out relevant self-monitoring (e.g., obese patients self-monitoring food intake). Of course, self-monitoring has to be set up appropriately and patients must be reinforced periodically for them to comply with the self-monitoring instructions. The final section of this chapter describes how to achieve this goal.

Self-monitoring headache activity serves two main functions. First, it leads to the generation of detailed information, relatively free from memory distortions, which contributes to the assessment process. Second, self-monitoring results in data that can serve as measures of treatment effectiveness. For some types of problems, self-monitoring can itself result in a reduction of the problem. Self-monitoring of cigarettes desired but not smoked decreases smoking, for example (McFall, 1970). It seems plausible that self-monitoring headache activity might lead to a reduction in headaches, because it should result in patients beginning to understand their headache problem better and consequently initiating changes. However, research has shown that self-monitoring on its own has little impact on headache activity (Blanchard et al., 1980; Holroyd & Penzien, 1986).

The two main types of self-monitoring used with headache sufferers are time sampling, where records of headache activity are completed at set times, and event sampling, where records of headache activity are completed according to the occurrence of some event (e.g., onset or offset of a headache).

Time Sampling

The main method used by headache researchers to assess treatment effectiveness is a headache diary in which patients periodically rate the intensity of their headaches. In addition to the headache ratings, the diaries usually require subjects to record medication taken for headaches; some require a record of all medication taken whether for headaches or for other reasons. Other variables recorded in such diaries include pain location (Bakal, 1982; Salkovskis, 1989; Thompson & Figueroa, 1983), activities (Bakal & Kaganov, 1976; Salkovskis, 1989), associated symptoms (Bakal, 1982; Thompson & Figueroa, 1983; Kewman & Roberts, 1980), impairment/disability from headache (Sargent, Walters, & Green, 1973; Kewman & Roberts, 1980), and situations (Bakal & Kaganov, 1976).

With respect to recording headache activity, systems have varied in terms of the rating scales used and how often the ratings are required. Scales have consisted of 3 points (e.g., Medina & Diamond, 1978), 4 points (e.g., Sargent, Walters, & Green, 1973), 6 points (e.g., Budzynski et al., 1973), 11 points (e.g., Haynes et al., 1975), 100 points (e.g., Chesney & Shelton, 1976), and visual analogue (Anciano, 1986). The points are defined in terms of intensity (e.g., slight, moderate) or impact of the headache on activities (e.g., a headache that can be ignored at times), or both. Ratings have been requested at the following frequencies: hourly (e.g., Budzynski et al., 1973), every 2 hours (e.g., Bakal, 1982), four times a day (breakfast, lunch, dinner, and bedtime) (e.g., Epstein & Abel, 1977), and daily (bedtime) (e.g., Thompson & Figueroa, 1983). Some systems require patients to rate their headache as it is at the time of rating; others ask for ratings pertaining to the period between the last rating and the current rating, or that day.

Headache diaries are usually kept on cards or notebooks that are small enough to be carried around easily. Patients generally record their ratings by placing crosses on graphs, although Bakal and colleagues use a different system in which patients record numbers indicating the location of their pain in selected boxes that indicate the intensity of their pain (Bakal, 1982; Bakal & Kaganov, 1976).

Collins and Thompson (1979) assessed the reliability of recording headache intensity four times a day by implementing three procedures to detect inaccurate recording. Their results were not very supportive of the reliability of self-monitoring data, as 40% of the subject sample were detected as being noncompliant in their recordings. The most common type of noncompliance involved subjects trying to recall pain levels at a later time rather than recording the levels using time-sampling procedures. On the other hand, as acknowledged by the authors, the study was carried out on a student sample only 17.7% of whom were experiencing headaches, so it is unclear whether their findings would generalize to a clinical population. Also, achieving a low rate of compliance in one study does not imply that a higher rate of compliance cannot be achieved using a different methodology. Nevertheless, this study provides an important warning against the uncritical use of self-monitoring and acceptance of the data it yields.

Blanchard, Andrasik, Neff, Jurish, and O'Keefe (1981) investigated the social validity of headache diaries by comparing improvement in headaches following treatment as assessed from diaries with improvement as assessed by significant others. The correlation between these two measures of change was .44 ($p < .002$).

The self-monitoring system that we have used in our research program and which I recommend for clinical use is the one devised by Budzynski et al. (1973). Patients are asked to keep records of their headaches and medication usage on 4" × 6" cards referred to as daily cards. The two sides of the daily card are shown in Figure 6.1.

On one side of the card, patients are required to record all medication consumed. They are asked to rate their headache intensity hourly on a 6-point scale throughout the waking day and to record the ratings on the other side of the card. The rating scale that I use is shown in Table 6.2. To help patients complete these diaries, they are given a set of written instructions, a copy of the rating scale, and a completed card as an example.

This system has a number of advantages over the alternatives. Recording headache activity hourly results in more information than recording less frequently. Frequent sampling is essential for recording headaches of short duration. Hourly recording gives the best opportunity for pursuing the follow-

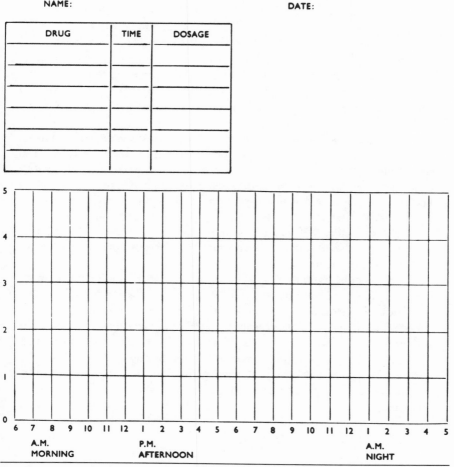

FIGURE 6.1. Daily card.

TABLE 6.2. Scale for Rating Headache Intensity

5 – An intense incapacitating headache
4 – A very severe headache which makes concentration difficult, but during which you could perform tasks of an undemanding nature
3 – A painful headache, but one during which you could continue at your job
2 – A headache that can be ignored at times
1 – A headache of a very low level type which enters awareness only at times when attention is devoted to it
0 – No headache

Adapted from Budzynski et al. (1973).

ing clinically significant issues: daily cycles in headache activity, the relationship between medication consumption and headache activity, and the frequency and duration of headaches. The only argument against hourly ratings is that they may create too much of a burden for patients. However, while patients usually say that the task is difficult and intrusive initially, because they must remember to keep the day's card with them and to complete the ratings on the hour, and they have to think carefully about which ratings to use, as the task becomes more of a habit, it becomes simpler and relatively effortless.

We have tried ratings at other frequencies. In our experience, ratings every 2 hours are unpopular with patients. It is easier for them to remember to record on the hour than to record every other hour. Recording ratings four times a day is less intrusive and easier to remember than hourly ratings because it is associated with daily events. Consequently, this frequency is worth considering for patients who do not suffer from brief headaches, particularly if other self-monitoring information is required. Daily ratings seem to offset the advantages of self-monitoring because they involve retrospective, global judgments.

The system I use only records headaches and medication consumption. Some of the information recorded by other systems is of limited value (e.g., pain location, associated symptoms). Other information is of greater significance (e.g., activities, situation), but I prefer to collect these data by other self-monitoring procedures as detailed in the next section. It is sometimes desirable to start the headache diaries before the first appointment, and they need to be completed over prolonged periods (before, during, and after treatment). Hence, these records must be straightforward for patients to complete.

Event Sampling

Event sampling has not been featured in the research literature but has been advocated in some clinically oriented publications. Diamond (1979) has published a copy of the headache record used at his headache clinic. Patients are requested to keep a record of their headaches using a form with the following seven columns: date, time onset–ending, severity of headache, psychic and physical factors, food and drink excesses, medication taken and dosage, and relief of headache. An interesting aspect of the record is a key printed on the back which largely reduces the patient's task to recording numbers or letters. The key includes two 10-point scales for rating severity and relief of headaches and coded lists of 21 psychic and physical factors and 21 food and drink excesses.

Holroyd and Andrasik (1982) advocate use of a record to be completed at the time of headache onset with the following six columns: time, situation, physical sensations, thoughts, feeling, and behavior.

Boudewyns (1982) has recommended a philosophy of assessment similar to the one outlined in this book. He emphasizes the need for evaluating events and experiences occurring just prior to, during, and following headaches, and suggests that these occurrences can be classified under the headings stimulus factors, organismic factors, and response factors. Patients are asked to complete a pain log divided into 10 columns. Column one is for recording the date and the next three columns are for recording stimulus factors: Time, Place, and Feeling State Thoughts Behavior. Four columns are devoted to organismic factors: Length of Time, Location, Intensity, and Description and Comment about Related Experience. The final two columns are for the response factors of Behavior in Response to Pain and Effect on Activities.

The event sampling system I have developed focuses on the time of most interest, that is, the time of changes in headache activity (P. R. Martin, 1983). Hence, this system parallels the functional analysis section of the PAHQ. Patients are asked to complete two types of cards: "change" and "control" cards. Change cards are designed to give detailed information about what patients are doing and how they are thinking and feeling at the time of headache change. They are intended to be used in conjunction with daily cards. A headache change is operationally defined as a headache beginning, a headache ending, or a headache changing in severity by 2 points or more on the headache intensity scale from 1 hour to the next, whether the headache increases or decreases in intensity. The change cards also measure 4″ × 6″, and the two sides of the cards are shown in Figure 6.2.

Headache ratings are completed using the 6-point scale shown in Table 6.2, and ratings of anxiety, depression, and stress are also completed using a 6-point scale (very severely, severely, moderately, slightly, very slightly, not at all). To help patients use these cards they are given a set of written in-structions, a copy of the rating scales, and a completed card as an example.

The control cards are designed to provide detailed information about what patients do and how they think and feel when free of headaches, so that this information can be compared with the same information collected at the time of headache changes. Patients are asked to complete a control card for each hour that they are headache free immediately after recording an hourly rating (of zero) on the daily cards, up to a maximum of four cards in a day. The two sides of the control card are shown in Figure 6.3.

Clinical Use of Self-Monitoring

Unlike the researcher, the clinician has the luxury of being able to individual-ize the self-monitoring task according to the needs of the particular patient. On the other hand, there are advantages to using a standardized system such as having record cards and instruction sheets available from first contact with

NAME: DATE: TIME:

PLACE CHANGE OCCURRED:

PEOPLE PRESENT:

HEADACHE CHANGE													
BEFORE							AFTER						
0	I	2	3	4	5	Ratings	0	I	2	3	4	5	
						Feelings							
0	I	2	3	4	5	Anxiety	0	I	2	3	4	5	
0	I	2	3	4	5	Depression	0	I	2	3	4	5	
						Thoughts							
0	I	2	3	4	5	Stress	0	I	2	3	4	5	
						Activities							
0	I	2	3	4	5	Stress	0	I	2	3	4	5	

FIGURE 6.2. Change card.

the patient. I tend to use the daily, change, and control cards with all the headache sufferers I see, but I sometimes introduce variations. I ask headache sufferers who believe that they experience two quite distinct types of headaches to record both types on the daily cards using crosses for one type of headache and circles for the other. I use the same system for patients with multiple pain problems (e.g., headaches and low back pain). If headaches are of brief duration (i.e., less than 1 hour), some form of event sampling is required whereby they record headaches as they occur. Such headaches are rare, however.

NAME:				DATE:			TIME:

PLACE OF RATING:

PEOPLE PRESENT:

Rating	0	1	2	3	4	5

Feelings

| Anxiety | 0 | 1 | 2 | 3 | 4 | 5 |
| Depression | 0 | 1 | 2 | 3 | 4 | 5 |

Thoughts

| Stress | 0 | 1 | 2 | 3 | 4 | 5 |

Activities

| Stress | 0 | 1 | 2 | 3 | 4 | 5 |

FIGURE 6.3. Control card.

An important point to consider is how long patients need to record their headaches prior to commencing treatment. As the majority of patients seen for treatment are female and a high proportion of female patients report that their headaches are worse during a particular phase of the menstrual cycle, it would seem that a 4-week baseline is necessary. This length of baseline is common in the headache research literature particularly for migraine samples. However, such an extended assessment record prior to treatment is difficult to implement in clinical practice, and fortunately the research literature suggests that it is unnecessary. Blanchard, Hillhouse, Appelbaum, and Jaccard (1987) assessed the adequacy of different lengths of baseline by correlating scores for baselines of 1, 2, or 3 weeks with scores from a 4-week baseline. Their analyses led them to recommend a 1-week baseline for clinical purposes with tension headache sufferers (2 weeks for research purposes) and a 2-week baseline for clinical purposes with migraine and combined headache sufferers (3 weeks for research purposes). I suggest that all patients be encouraged to complete the daily cards for 2 weeks prior to commencing active treatment strategies (i.e., not including the educational component of treatment).

For the successful establishment of self-monitoring, three conditions need to be met: (1) patients must understand and be able to recall the task required of them, (2) the task must not be too intrusive or onerous to carry out, and (3) patients must be convinced of the relevance and importance of completing the task. To ensure comprehension and recall, instructions should be given verbally and in written form. I often get patients to complete a card retrospectively in my presence for the last day they experienced a headache, for practice purposes. However, if this strategy is adopted it is important to emphasize that patients should not complete the cards retrospectively in the future.

Using the three types of self-monitoring cards described earlier does not seem to make the task too intrusive or burdensome. I do not start patients on all three types of cards at the same time, however, because this tends to overload them. I usually introduce the change and control cards about 2 weeks after patients have started using the daily cards. I ask patients to use the daily cards for 2 weeks before treatment, throughout the treatment period, and for 2 weeks after treatment. The change and control cards are used more selectively, usually for one, or two 2-week periods.

The relevance and importance of the task can be communicated in a number of ways. One is to carefully explain the purpose of the cards and to emphasize that they are a critical component of the assessment process. A more indirect approach is to imply their importance by the way in which the task is set up. For example, I arrange for each patient to be given a set of 20 daily cards, an instruction sheet including a rating scale, and a completed card as an example; all these materials are placed in a folder with the patient's name typed on it. Instructions for the other types of cards can subsequently be added to this folder. Patients need periodic reinforcement to continue with self-monitoring. Typically this involves collecting the previous week's cards at the beginning of each session, checking whether any problems in recording were experienced, and praising the patient's efforts.

There are many different ways to extract information from self-monitoring records. Dalton (1973) has advocated using "frequency charts" which comprise tables consisting of 12 columns, one for each month of the year, and 31 rows, one for each possible day of the month. An "H" or "h" is placed in the appropriate box to denote a headache (upper case for a severe headache and lower case for a mild headache) and a "P" for period. If self-monitoring is continued for a long time, this type of chart is good for exposing certain types of relationships such as associations between headaches and menstruation.

In clinical practice, I calculate from each daily card a daily average headache rating (i.e., a sum of all the ratings divided by the number of ratings). I transcribe onto forms the following from the cards: date (asterisks are placed against potentially significant days such as weekends), average rating (asterisks are used to highlight high ratings), and medication consumption (a pill count of all drugs taken for the headaches). From the daily average ratings and medication consumption data, weekly averages are calculated and graphed.

A combination of inspection of the cards, forms, and graphs enables evaluation of the daily, weekly, and monthly cycles; the relationship between headaches and medication consumption; and the effect of treatment on headache activity and medication usage. Additional analysis of ratings can be used to clarify patterns. For example, if headache activity appears to be less frequent on weekends than on weekdays, a simple calculation will support the impression.

7

Specialized Methods for Assessing Headache Phenomena, Antecedents, and Consequences

Headache Phenomena

Headaches and Associated Symptoms

The major methods for assessing headaches and associated symptoms—questionnaires, interviewing, and self-monitoring—were reviewed in the previous chapter. There is one additional approach to headache assessment that is also worth discussing. Headache researchers have been criticized on the grounds of viewing pain as a unidimensional phenomenon varying only in intensity (Allen & Weinmann, 1982). In contrast, the pain literature has acknowledged for many years that the pain experience includes at least two interacting components: (1) a sensory component, which includes attributes like intensity, location, and quality; and (2) a reactive component, which includes a person's emotional reaction to the pain, fears about what the pain signals, and concerns about his or her ability to cope with pain in a socially acceptable manner (Beecher, 1959).

To assess the unique qualities of different pain phenomena, Melzack developed the McGill Pain Questionnaire (MPQ) (Melzack, 1975). The MPQ consists of 78 pain descriptors divided into three major classes (sensory, affective, and evaluative) as well as a pain intensity scale. It takes about 5 minutes to complete and studies have shown it to have acceptable reliability and validity (Melzack, 1983).

The MPQ has been used with headache sufferers, although not extensively. Allen and Weinmann (1982) investigated whether the MPQ had a role in headache diagnosis. These investigators found no differences between migraineurs and tension headache sufferers on the sensory and evaluative dimensions but a significant difference on the affective dimension. The affective dimension measures emotional discomfort and migraineurs scored higher on this variable. I used the MPQ as an outcome measure in one of my treatment studies to evaluate whether the two treatments affected the three dimensions differentially (Martin et al., 1989). Results on this scale paralleled the headache diary findings. Other studies have used the MPQ as a measure against which to compare other measures of headache experience (e.g., Philips, 1989; Demjen et al., 1990; Penzien et al., 1985; Lacroix & Barbaree, 1990).

Tursky (1976) developed a "pain perception profile" for measuring the reactive as well as the sensory component of pain based on the MPQ. Andrasik, Blanchard, Ahles, Pallmeyer, and Barron (1981) found that Tursky's intensity adjectives correlated highly with the traditional numerical ratings whereas all correlations involving the affective adjectives were significantly lower in magnitude. In a second study by these researchers using Tursky's scale, they found that the reactive dimension discriminated between headache and nonheadache individuals rather than the intensity dimension (Blanchard, Andrasik, Arena, & Teders, 1982).

A third instrument composed of pain descriptors, the Headache Scale, was developed by Jahanshahi, Hunter, and Philips (1986). This scale also measures a sensory and affective component of pain. Administration of the Headache Scale to classical and common migraineurs and tension headache sufferers revealed quantitative but not qualitative differences between the groups.

Psychophysiological Mechanisms

If treatment involves biofeedback training, psychophysiological assessment pretreatment is mandatory. However, this book does not advocate biofeedback training because the evidence as reviewed in Chapter 5 suggests that EMG biofeedback training is associated with poor long-term maintenance, and other forms of biofeedback training are not superior to alternatives that do not require special equipment.

Turpin (1991) has argued strongly for including psychophysiological measurement at all stages of behavioral assessment; Haynes, Falkin, and Sexton-Radek (1989) have documented that the number of articles using psychophysiological measurement rose from around 1% in 1965 to about 40% in the 1980s in two leading behavior therapy journals. On the other hand, evidence reviewed in Chapter 3 demonstrates that, currently, the psychophysiological mechanisms of headaches are not clear, raising questions about which variables should be measured. Also, the reliability of psychophysiological assessment tends to be low, particularly for the variables that seem to be most relevant to headaches such as temporal BVP and hand temperature (Arena, Blanchard, Andrasik, Cotch, & Myers, 1983). I have discussed elsewhere why psychophysiological contributions to headache research have so far not fulfilled their potential (Johnston & Martin, 1991).

On balance, there seems little to be gained from incorporating psychophysiological measurement into psychological assessment procedures for headache sufferers in clinical practice. Hence, this topic is not pursued further here. For readers who do wish to carry out psychophysiological assessment, the general texts by Martin and Venables (1980), Coles, Donchin, and Porges (1986), and Turpin (1989) are recommended. Chapters on this topic have been written by Sturgis and Arena (1984) and Raczynski, Ray, and McCarthy (1991); methodological critiques of psychophysiological studies of headaches can be found in Andrasik, Blanchard, Arena, Saunders, and Barron (1982) and Raczynski and Thompson (1983).

Antecedents

Immediate Factors

The previous chapter reviewed some procedures for exploring the immediate antecedents of headaches. Hence, most questionnaires, including the PAHQ, include questions about precipitating and aggravating factors. Also, some of the self-monitoring procedures discussed the collection of information on antecedent factors (Martin, 1983; Diamond, 1979; Boudewyns, 1982).

A number of self-monitoring techniques have been developed for studying the relationship between stress and headaches. Levor et al. (1986) designed a diary system that involved subjects completing records three times a day. Headache symptoms were recorded, as were upsetting or stressful events and various emotional states. The diary included both preprinted common stressors, for example, "encounter with family/friend" and "time pressure," and idiosyncratic stressors identified by the individual at interview or on the Hassles Scales (HS) (Kanner, Coyne, Schaefer, & Lazarus, 1981) as being personally upsetting. These latter stressors were written into spaces in the diary, and individuals indicated by checkmarks whether events or feelings had occurred since the previous response time.

Kohler and Haimerl (1990) and Mosley et al. (1990) have asked individuals to complete stress questionnaires at the end of each day in addition to monitoring headaches. The questionnaire used by Kohler and Haimerl also contained items about menstrual cycle, alcohol consumption, and duration of sleep during the previous night.

A number of researchers have evaluated negative affect as an immediate antecedent of headaches by asking individuals to rate mood on scales (usually visual analogue) three times a day (Harrigan et al., 1984), two times a day (Harvey & Hay, 1984), or once a day (Arena et al., 1984). I have explored the same association using an event-sampling procedure rather than a time-sampling approach (Martin et al., 1988). In this study, patients were asked to complete a Profile of Mood States (POMS) (McNair & Lorr, 1982) at the end of specified headache days and headache-free days for comparative purposes. The POMS is a 72-item inventory designed to measure six mood states.

Dietary factors as precipitants of headaches have been studied by requesting individuals to complete "attack forms" immediately following recovery from a migraine (Dalton, 1973, 1975). The form records all food and drink consumed during the 24 hours immediately prior to an attack, together with other potential triggers under headings such as, Did you have any special worry, overwork or shock? and What had you done during the day (normal work, unusual activity, extra tired)?

The self-monitoring approaches to collecting information about the immediate antecedents of headaches are useful because they provide information that is more detailed and less biased by memory than simply asking patients about headache triggers. For example, although headaches are associated with a wide range of negative emotions, for individual sufferers the headaches may be associated with specific emotions (Martin et al., 1988). To illustrate this point, in my research on the relationship between headaches and the six mood states measured by the POMS, correlations for one subject ranged from −.06 with anxiety to −.61 with depression, for another they varied from .03 with hostility to −.53 with anxiety, and for another from .02 with depression to −.61 with unsureness. This type of data is useful for clinicians because it has implications for management.

Another option for clinicians is to carry out behavioral experiments that clarify relationships. It is common for patients to report associations for which the basis is quite unclear. For example, it may be noted that headaches are worse on weekends. If the observation is accurate (which can be verified via inspection of headache diaries), there are many possible explanations, including the following: (1) weekends are more stressful than weekdays for some reason (e.g., family conflicts), (2) weekends are less stressful and the headaches represent a "letdown" phenomenon or poststress relaxation, (3) the sufferer stays in bed longer, (4) breakfast is delayed, resulting in low blood sugar levels, (5) there are differences in diet, (6) there are differences in activities (e.g., activities may not be viewed as stressful but may involve exertion and fatigue), and (7) there are differences in environment (e.g., spending more or less time out of doors). Some possibilities can be eliminated by additional questions, but usually several explanations remain. If the association seems important (e.g., the effect is relatively substantial), it can be explored by designing behavioral experiments such as encouraging sufferers to follow weekday sleep and eating patterns throughout the weekend to assess whether these factors are significant.

Although I strongly advocate the behavioral experiment approach, a warning is necessary. Patients' reports of the effect of stimuli or events on their pain should be evaluated cautiously rather than automatically accepted at face value. A few examples of experiences from clinical research studies illustrate this point. A patient who had participated in a trial of physiotherapy for low back pain (Martin, Rose, Nichols, Russell, & Hughes, 1986) returned to see me 12 months later reporting that we had cured her problem but that she had recently tripped on stairs provoking a reoccurrence. She explained that we had eliminated a chronic pain problem which had incapacitated her and prevented her from working for over 20 years, while all other health professionals (orthodox and heterodox) had failed. She praised our treatment, which she wished to resume, but when we checked our records we found that she had been in the attention–placebo control group (untuned ultrasound and untuned short-wave diathermy).

In a contrasting example, I recently supervised a study investigating whether chocolate could precipitate headaches (Mazzella, 1992). One subject dropped out because of the headache he experienced following consumption of the first sample, a headache unprecedented in its severity. The sample was a placebo. Another subject took part in a study that employed a pain *induction* (nocebo) procedure (Martin, Marie, & Nathan, 1992) and reported that his long-standing headache problem was cured following participation.

Setting Factors

A number of questionnaires can contribute to the assessment process of headaches that seem to be triggered or aggravated by stress. One question raised by a stress–headache link pertains to the sources of stressors in the individual's life. Life-event inventories or structured interviews can be used for this purpose, such as the Rating Scale for Life Events (Paykel, Prusoff, & Uhlnhuth, 1971), the Social Readjustment Rating Scale (Holmes & Rahe, 1967), and the List of Recent Experiences (Henderson, Byrne, & Duncan-Jones, 1981). These questionnaires have had limited success, however, in discriminating headache sufferers from headache-free individuals (see Chapter 4). More useful instruments are the HS (Kanner et al., 1981) and the Perceived Stress Scale (PSS) (Cohen, Kamark, & Mermelstein, 1983). The HS consists of 117 items that reflect annoying daily problems that have occurred in the previous month rather than major life events. The scale is designed to collect information not only about the number of hassles individuals experience but also about their perceived severity. The PSS is a 14-item measure of the degree to which situations in one's life are appraised as stressful.

Holm et al. (1986) demonstrated that headache sufferers were disadvantaged relative to controls in terms of both stress appraisal and coping processes. An evaluation of such processes in individuals suffering from stress-related headaches would be appropriate, but the scales used in this study have not been published. Information is provided regarding the scales, however. Coping appraisal was measured by an inventory adapted from an Attribution Questionnaire (Hammen & Mayol, 1982). Coping strategies were assessed by a 76-item inventory based on the Ways of Coping Scale (Lazarus & Folkman, 1984).

Another relevant factor to assess for stress-related headaches is perceived social support. We have found that the Interview Schedule for Social Interaction (ISSI) (Henderson, Duncan-Jones, Byrne, & Scott, 1980), the Social Support Questionnaire (SSQ) (Sarason, Levine, Basham, & Sarason, 1983), and the Interpersonal Support Evaluation List (ISEL) (Cohen, Mermelstein, Kamarck, & Hoberman, 1985) all discriminate between headache sufferers and headache-free controls. The SSQ and ISEL are preferable to the ISSI because they are questionnaires while the ISSI is a structured interview. The SSQ consists of 27 items and assesses perceived availability of social support and satisfaction with perceived support. The ISEL includes 40 items and was developed in order to measure the availability of four different functions that an individual's support network might provide: appraisal or informational support, esteem or emotional support, belonging or instrumental support, and tangible support.

A common source of stress in headache sufferers is the marital relationship, so instruments that measure marital discord, such as the DAS (Spanier, 1976), can be useful.

Because headaches are often triggered by negative emotions, anxiety and depressive symptoms can be considered setting factors for headaches. Hence, measures of emotional symptoms such as the BDI and the STAI are appropriate for assessing setting factors. These instruments were discussed in Chapter 6.

Onset Factors

In exploring onset antecedents, one first needs information about when the headache problem began. Sometime there are two important dates because the headaches may have begun at one time but become significantly worse at another.

Pinpointing the onset period can be difficult since onset may have been gradual and may have occurred a long time ago. Also, follow-up questions often reveal that the initial response to "When did the headaches begin?" is apparently inaccurate. Either patients overestimate chronicity by responding on the basis of the first headache they can remember rather than when the headaches became a significant problem, or they underestimate as a consequence of forgetting their early experience of problem headaches.

The most direct approach to investigating onset antecedents is to ask patients to identify the events or circumstances that they think may have contributed to the onset of the headaches. Question 24.3 in the PAHQ does this by starting with the onset factors identified in the research literature. An alternative approach is to inquire about changes that took place around the identified time of headache onset. Life-event inventories such as the Social Readjustment Rating Scale (Holmes & Rahe, 1967) can provide cues to aid recall.

Predisposing Factors

One method of exploring a predisposition to developing headaches is to investigate family history of headaches (question 25 in the PAHQ). It should be noted, however, that asking patients about family incidence of headaches does not always yield accurate information (Waters, 1971).

Personality inventories can be administered to explore personality characteristics that may make an individual susceptible to headaches. An MMPI can be given, for example, to assess whether the individual fits the conversion V pattern, although the evidence relating headaches to personality profiles such as these is mixed (see Chapter 4). Administration of an MMPI can serve other functions also (e.g., screening for psychopathology) and as a predictor of treatment outcome (see Chapter 5).

I do not particularly recommend the MMPI as a routine component of headache assessment in clinical practice, but I have found the Framingham Type A scale (Haynes, Levine, Scotch, Feinleib, & Kannel, 1978) to be quite useful. A high proportion of headaches are related to stress, but there are many different pathways and processes linking "disease" to psychobiological stress responses (Steptoe, 1991). The stress causing headaches may result from an individual's being overcommitted and trying to achieve too much, or it may result from an individual's becoming morbidly preoccupied by his or her pain and spending too much time ruminating about the headaches (Martin, Nathan, & Milech, 1987). The former, and larger, group tends to be Type A's and the latter group Type B's, hence providing the rationale for administering a Type A questionnaire. The distinction is important because it has clear implications for management. Because both types of headaches are stress related, techniques that target the stress response, such as relaxation training, are likely to be useful for both groups. But Type A's need to be encouraged to reduce their commitments and Type B's need to be encouraged to become more active.

Consequences

Immediate Reactions

The immediate reactions of headache sufferers and significant others to headaches need careful assessment in order to identify maladaptive responses. Five hypotheses pertaining to maladaptive reactions were discussed in Chapters 1 and 4: reinforcement, avoidance behavior, exacerbating antecedents, enhancing pain perception, and drug-induced.

Interviewing is the main method for collecting information relevant to the reinforcement hypothesis, and a number of questions on the PAHQ are included for this purpose. Additional questions may need to be asked when reinforcement mechanisms seem to be a possibility.

The reinforcement hypothesis is difficult to assess. A positive reinforcer is any event, behavior, privilege, or material object that will increase the probability of occurrence of any behavior upon which it is contingent; a negative reinforcer is any event whose contingent withdrawal increases the rate of performance of a response (Rimm & Masters, 1979). Responses to headaches such as spousal reassurance and consolation, or getting medication, seem likely to be positive reinforcers, whereas responses to headaches involving termination of aversive conditions such as stressful work or family situations seem likely to be negative reinforcers. The word *likely* is used, however, because it is only possible to be certain that an event is a reinforcer if it can be observed that the contingent presentation of the speculated reinforcer does, indeed, affect the behavior of the person in question.

Fordyce (1976) presented a detailed description of how to assess whether pain behaviors are influenced by the consequences that follow them. Whereas this book is a seminal contribution to the field, the logic of some of his suggestions is debatable, and the focus of his work has been on low back pain rather than on headaches. Although there are clear parallels between these two pain populations, there are also major differences. For example, back pain begins with some form of organic pathology, which may or may not resolve, but this is not the case for migraines or tension headaches.

In assessing whether headaches are maintained by social reinforcement, the first question to answer is whether others in the vicinity of the headache sufferer can reliably discriminate headache and headache-free states. If they cannot, there is no opportunity for social reinforcement. Even answering this question is not a trivial task because social desirability response factors may encourage headache sufferers to answer in terms of not "burdening" others. Also, the cues that signal that a headache is being experienced are often subtle ones, such as changes in activities or facial appearance rather than verbal reports.

Deciding whether a response to headaches constitutes a reinforcer is difficult. Even reactions by spouses characterized by negative emotions such as frustration and anger can serve as positive reinforcers because they may reassure the patient that the spouse is still aware of the problem, or the sufferer may delight in causing the spouse distress. In contrast, even if headaches are followed by events that appear to have considerable value for the sufferer, this does not necessarily imply that the headaches are maintained by their consequences.

Fordyce (1976) suggests that the critical factor is the consistency of the reaction by the spouse rather than the nature of his or her reactions. Certainly if the response by spouses is highly variable it seems unlikely that learning will occur. As behavior can be maintained by partial reinforcement schedules, however, some degree of inconsistency, particularly once the response has been acquired, would not seem incompatible with operant factors contributing to headaches.

Turning to the avoidance behavior hypothesis, various versions of the PBC can be used to collect relevant information. Philips and Hunter (1981) published the original 19-item form of this scale which was also used by Anciano (1986) and Appelbaum et al. (1988). Philips and Jahanshahi (1986) extended the PBC to 49 items and established the reliability and validity of the new scale. Factor analysis of the responses to this questionnaire resulted in 13 independent behavioral factors of pain behavior (see Chapter 4). The authors argued that using a scaling procedure derived from the factor analysis, consisting of summing responses on items loading on specific factors, enables an assessment of the specific types of pain behavior used by individuals which can then be used to plan a behavioral management program. They offer as an example that for patients with high verbal and nonverbal complaint factor scores, the issue of secondary gain and the importance of environmental modification would feature highly in a treatment program; in contrast, patients with high social avoidance scores would need a different behavioral emphasis.

With respect to the exacerbating antecedents hypothesis, the HAQ (Bakal, 1982) provides useful information concerning thoughts and feelings experienced at headache onset, and therefore helps evaluate whether individuals whose headaches are precipitated by stress and negative affect react to their headaches with negative emotion, thereby completing a vicious cycle. Researchers have developed variations of this questionnaire (Philips, 1989; Demjen et al., 1990), but the variations do not differ substantially from the original version, and unlike the original version, full details of the revised scales have not been published. The HAQ consists of 48 items to which individuals respond using 4-point Likert scales. Individuals are asked to complete the questionnaire immediately following their next severe headache attack. Penzien et al. (1985) present evidence testifying to the discriminant and construct validity of the HAQ.

The enhancing pain perception hypothesis suggests that reactions to pain characterized by anxiety, focusing on the pain, and loss of sense of control over pain will exacerbate the pain experience. The methods of assessing whether pain is associated with these affective and cognitive responses overlap those already discussed. Links with anxiety can be explored by self-monitoring with either mood rating scales or the POMS. Associations with focus of attention and sense of control can be assessed with questionnaires such as the HAQ.

The drug-induced hypothesis is best explored by the self-monitoring of medication intake, as discussed in Chapter 6. Records of medication intake need to be evaluated for use of ergotamine tartrate, analgesics, and drugs with headaches as a side effect. Saper (1987) has suggested that ingesting ergotamine on 2 or 3 days per week or more can induce daily or almost daily headaches of a migraine type. The IHS classification system includes three criteria for "analgesics abuse headache": (1) greater than or equal to 50 g of aspirin a month or equivalent of other mild analgesics, (2) greater than or equal to 100 tablets a month of analgesics combined with barbiturates or other nonnarcotic compounds, and (3) one or more narcotic analgesics.

Long-Term Effects

Questions 23.1 and 23.2 in the PAHQ enquire about the long-term effects of headaches. Caution needs to be exercised in exploring long-term consequences. Individuals often answer that headaches have stopped their engaging in certain activities, but a follow-up question reveals that they never engaged in these activities prior to developing the headache problem.

A number of questionnaires can be used for evaluating the long-term effects of chronic headaches. Instruments that have been employed for this purpose in the research literature include the CPQ (Lacroix & Barbaree, 1990), the NHP (Jenkinson, 1990; Jenkinson & Fitzpatrick, 1990), and the Sickness Impact Profile (Carlsson et al., 1990). Of these questionnaires, the CPQ developed by Monks and Taenzer (1983) is particularly useful. Parenthetically, these authors also provide a review of alternative pain assessment questionnaires.

The CPQ is designed to be a comprehensive pain assessment questionnaire and is composed of two complementary parts, the Patient Questionnaire and the Interviewer Guide. The Patient Questionnaire is mailed to the patient prior to the first clinic appointment. The interviewer reviews the Patient Questionnaire, clarifies responses as necessary, and adds more complex or private inquiries such as those in the Interviewer Guide.

The CPQ is long, not specific to headaches, and overlaps considerably with items on headache questionnaires such as the PAHQ. Hence, if used for headache sufferers within the functional framework advocated in this book, it would be appropriate to use a much abbreviated version of the scale. Question 10 in the Patient Questionnaire, which inquires into the effects of pain on work, finances, legal proceedings, leisure, sleep, weight/diet, and habits, is the most relevant here.

Assessment Summary

Many different assessment techniques were discussed in this chapter and the preceding chapter. Rather than provide a prescriptive list of approaches, techniques will be divided into four categories. The first category consists of techniques that are strongly recommended for use with all headache sufferers.

TABLE 7.1. Recommended Assessment Techniques and Alternatives

Strongly recommended	Alternatives
Semistructured interview	
PAHQ (Appendix 4) Begin in Session 1 and continue into Session 2 or 3	History form (Blanchard & Andrasik, 1985)
Self-monitoring	
Daily cards (Figure 6.1) Begin before or immediately after Session 1 and continue throughout treatment and for 2 weeks after treatment	Diaries with headache ratings four times a day (Epstein & Abel, 1977)
Change and control cards (Figures 6.2 & 6.3) Begin at least 2 weeks after starting daily cards and continue for at least 2 weeks	Headache record (Diamond, 1979) Pain log (Boudewyns, 1982) Record of events (Holroyd & Andrasik, 1982)
Questionnaires	
BDI (Beck et al., 1961) Ask patients to complete before or after Session 1	Self-rating Depression Scale (Zung, 1965)
STAI (Spielberger et al., 1970) As for BDI	Taylor Manifest Anxiety Scale (Taylor, 1953)

The second category consists of techniques that are alternatives to the first category. Techniques in categories one and two are listed in Table 7.1, together with information pertaining to when category one techniques should be applied.

The third category consists of techniques that are worth considering in particular circumstances. The final category is techniques that could be used but are not strongly advocated. Some are alternatives to those in the third category, but others provide different assessment information. Techniques in categories three and four are listed in Table 7.2 together with information pertaining to when they are appropriate.

TABLE 7.2. Supplementary Assessment Techniques

Worth considering	Possibilities
Headaches and associated symptoms	
If wish to take a multidimensional view of pain:	
MPQ (Melzack, 1975)	Pain Perception Profile (Tursky, 1976)
	Headache Scale (Jahanshahi et al., 1986)
Immediate antecedents	
If wish to pursue stress as a trigger of headaches:	
Stress diaries (Levor et al., 1986)	Daily stress inventory (Mosley et al., 1990)
	Daily stress questionnaire (Kohler & Haimerl, 1990)
If wish to pursue negative affect as a trigger of headaches:	
POMS (McNair & Lorr, 1982)	Mood scales (Harrigan et al., 1984)
	Visual analogue scales (Harvey & Hay, 1984)
If wish to pursue dietary factors as a trigger of headaches:	
Attack forms (Dalton, 1973, 1975)	
If wish to clarify nature of observed associations:	
Behavioral experiments	
Setting antecedents	
If wish to pursue sources of stress:	
HS (Kanner et al., 1981)	PSS (Cohen, Kamark, & Mermelstein, 1983)
If wish to assess social support as a moderator of stress:	
SSQ (Sarason et al., 1983)	ISEL (Cohen et al., 1985)
If wish to assess marital satisfaction as a potential source of stress:	
DAS (Spanier, 1976)	

(continued)

TABLE 7.2. (Continued)

Worth considering	Possibilities

Onset antecedents

Aid to recall of significant events at time of headache onset:

Social Readjustment Rating Scale (Holmes &
  Rahe, 1967)

Predisposing antecedents

If wish to investigate personality characteristics as predispositional factors:

Framingham Type A scale (Haynes et al.,   MMPI
  1978)

Immediate reactions

Useful questionnaire for avoidance behavior and reinforcement hypotheses:

PBC (Philips & Jahanshahi, 1986)

Useful questionnaire for exacerbating antecedents and enhancing pain perception hypotheses:

HAQ (Bakal, 1982)

Long-term effects

CPQ (Monks & Taenzer, 1983) (abbreviated version)	NHP (Hunt, McEwen, & McKenna, 1986) Sickness Impact Profile (Bergner, Bobbitt, Carter, & Gilson, 1981)

8

Case Examples of Psychological Assessment from a Functional Perspective

The following two cases were assessed according to the functional model and procedures recommended in this book. The treatment of these two cases is discussed in the final chapter.

Case I: Clare

Clare was a 32-year-old married housewife with three young sons, referred to me by her family practitioner for headaches which had a history dating back 16 years. She had lived locally all her life except for two short periods. She had been educated at a private school followed by training as a primary school teacher. She described herself as a practicing Roman Catholic but not a regular church attender. She did not smoke cigarettes and only drank an occasional glass of wine with a meal.

Clare had been married for 7 years to Jim, age 30. Jim had trained as a civil engineer but was working for a company that designed office interiors. Clare became pregnant after her first term as a primary teacher and had not worked outside the home since. Clare and Jim had three sons ages 6 years, 3 years, and 4 months. Clare had two older sisters. Both sisters and her parents lived locally. Clare described her family as very "closely knit" and volunteered that Jim thought that they were too close.

Clare started taking a contraceptive pill at the time of her marriage but discontinued after 3 months because it made her headaches worse and resulted in her feeling nauseous. She tried a different brand of pill after giving birth to her first child but it also aggravated her headaches and made her feel unwell. Since then she had used an intrauterine device.

Clare scored 14 on the BDI (long form) which placed her in the mild depression category. Her scores on the STAI placed her on the 75th percentile for state anxiety and the 71st percentile for trait anxiety.

Clare could differentiate two types of headaches although type II was clearly a progression from type I. All headaches began with an uncomfortable feeling in the back of her neck. Clare responded to her headaches by taking medication and this sometimes resolved the headaches. On other occasions they developed into type II headaches. Clare described type I headaches as an aching, nagging pain, whereas type II headaches were more intense and were experienced as thumping. Both types of headaches were localized in the same region of the head. The pain began in the neck, sometimes on the right and sometimes on the left. The pain could radiate to any position in the head but settled more on the right than the left and was often focused behind the eye.

The only prodromal symptom was the neck discomfort. Symptoms associated with the type II headaches included nausea and vomiting had occurred in the past, but not in recent years. Clare described her headaches as almost a daily occurrence, an observation confirmed by self-monitoring. Inspection of the daily cards revealed that her headaches varied in duration from 1 to 6 hours with as many as four episodes occurring in a single day. Headache intensity ratings ranged from 1 to 3 on the 6-point scale (see Table 6.2).

Clare had been seen by a neurologist shortly before referral, who completed a general physical and neurological examination. The neurologist had also organized neck and back X rays and a cranial CAT scan. None of these assessments revealed significant pathology. Clare had received treatment from the following health practitioners: physiotherapist, dietitian, osteopath, chiropractor, and acupuncturist. She reported that none of these treatments had helped her. Clare's family practitioner had given her Dixarit and she had tried Sandomigran, but these medications brought no relief.

Self-monitoring over a 2-week period before the commencement of treatment revealed that Clare took medication for headaches on all but 2 days. She consumed up to three Mersyndol (450 mgs each), two Disprin (300 mgs each), and three Aspro Clear (300 mgs each) in a day. She had also taken Mogadon and Pensig.

In terms of the IHS classification system, Clare's type I headaches fulfilled the criteria for chronic tension-type headaches, and the type II headaches fulfilled the criteria for migraine without aura. From a functional perspective, the hypothesized controlling variables of Clare's headaches are shown in Figure 8.1. With respect to the factors that precipitated or aggra-

→

FIGURE 8.1. Functional model of Clare's headaches.

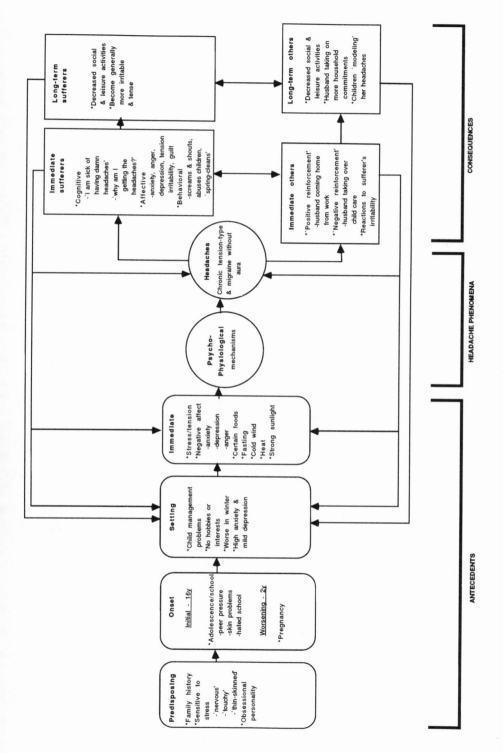

135

vated headaches, questioning combined with inspection of the change and control cards revealed the following: Clare emphasized stress and tension. The examples of stressors that she offered were "kids being obnoxious," "racing round doing things," and "hassles in the home." Anxiety, depression, and anger appeared consistently on the change cards prior to a headache's beginning or becoming significantly more intense, but they appeared infrequently on the control cards. Other immediate antecedents elicited by questioning indicated certain foods (e.g., nuts)—although she had been avoiding them for some time thus obscuring the observation—fasting (she believed she had to eat regularly), cold wind, heat, and strong sunlight.

One life-style factor that seemed to make Clare vulnerable to headaches was her difficulties in managing her three children. She frequently described her sons as wild and obnoxious. She said that they threw temper tantrums and were very demanding. She reported that they had problems in socializing and she tried not to take them out with her. She stated that she got sick of apologizing for them. A second, related setting factor was that Clare had no hobbies or interests. She indicated that her time was totally consumed by headaches and children. Because she had suffered from headaches since her teens, it was difficult to identify any hobbies and interests prior to her headaches and children.

Clare reported that her headaches were worse in winter than at other times of the year. This could reflect meteorological conditions (e.g., cold wind), behavioral factors such as doing more cooking (her husband often cooked the food on a barbecue in the summer), or the children's spending more time indoors in winter. Clare's high trait anxiety and mild depression could also be considered setting factors, because the negative emotions and depression could trigger headaches.

Clare had suffered from nausea, vomiting, and occasional headaches for as long as she could remember, but the headaches first became a real problem when she was in high school, which she hated. She considered the church school she attended to be very narrow, and an institution that did not allow students to have opinions of their own. Errors were unacceptable. Clare also felt very conscious of perceived peer group pressure at school. She believed that she had to "be like everyone else," and had to have the "right" boyfriend. Adolescent skin problems had distressed her considerably. She described this period of her life as "pretty horrific."

Clare's headaches had become significantly worse in the 12 months prior to referral, a period in which she began her third pregnancy. It was unclear whether the exacerbation related to hormonal factors or to the additional pressures that evolve from pregnancy.

Clare had a strong family history of headaches. Her mother and maternal grandmother suffered from headaches, although their headaches had improved as they grew older. Also, her elder sister suffered from debilitating headaches. Various aspects of Clare's personality seemed to predispose her to developing headaches or other stress-related disorders. She was very sensitive to stress and described herself as "nervous," "touchy," and "thin-skinned." She volunteered that little things upset her and that she had no patience. In addition, Clare was highly obsessional about her household. She said that she was "very strong on cleanliness," and expected her home always to be neat and tidy.

As for the consequences of headaches, Clare's immediate responses to headaches were assessed by questioning combined with information from the change and control cards. Her cognitive responses to a headache developing included the following: Damn this headache, I hope it goes away soon. This headache is going to make the morning even more unbearable. Why am I getting this headache? I hate having headaches. Affective responses included anxiety, anger, depression, tension, irritability, and guilt. Clare's behavioral reactions to headaches included screaming and shouting at the family and verbally abusing the children. Also, she would react to a headache, or even the belief that one was going to develop, by spring cleaning her home, because she felt that a headache would incapacitate her and prevent her from fulfilling her household responsibilities.

Clare reported that she tried not to tell others about her headaches because "they think you are neurotic." She did indicate, however, that both her husband and her mother could recognize when she had a headache. She reported that they would say, "Have you got a headache?" in a manner that she interpreted as accusatory.

If Clare developed an intense headache while Jim was at work, she would contact him and he would return home. She said that he "wouldn't say a lot, just look," and "he would have to take over the kids, but would be lousy about it." Clare believed that he would go out of his way to create a mess in the house to communicate to her his displeasure with her headaches. Clare's irritability, screaming, and shouting, resulted in Jim's retaliating in kind.

With respect to the long-term effects of headaches, Clare had adopted a life-style that was dominated by headaches. Her headaches appeared to have resulted in decreased social and leisure activities for her and her family, although it was difficult to determine whether the limited socializing was linked to the headaches or to problems with the children, or reflected other factors such as personality characteristics. Clare believed that the headaches had affected her personality by making her generally more irritable and tense. One implication of the headaches for Jim was that he had to accept more household commitments, in particular, looking after the children. Jim had suggested that Clare's verbal abuse was making the children "neurotic," and Clare believed that the children had learned that the way to avoid undesirable activities was to say that they had a headache.

Regarding headache mechanisms, one can see a clear theme of stress and negative affect running through the antecedent factors of Clare's headaches. Clare is an individual predisposed to developing headaches and stress-related problems, and she began to suffer from headaches during a period of high stress. Clare lived a life-style dominated by headaches and problems with her children, with no space for activities that would result in positive feelings such as pleasure and sense of accomplishment. However, her headaches could be triggered by a number of factors, in addition to stress and negative feelings, which fall into the categories of consummatory stimuli (certain foods, fasting) and meteorological conditions (cold wind, heat, strong sunlight).

Some of the reactions of her and her husband seemed likely to be maladaptive. Jim's coming home from work and taking over the child care might constitute positive and negative reinforcement, respectively. A number of vicious cycles seemed to operate. Negative affect could precipitate headaches which would result in further negative affect. Stress could trigger headaches, which would result in family rows, which would in turn elevate stress levels. Spring cleaning in response to a headache's beginning or being anticipated would guarantee that the headache occurred ("racing round doing things" was reported to be a precipitant). Screaming and shouting at the children exacerbated Clare's difficulties in relating positively and constructively to them.

Clare responded to her headaches by focusing on them and becoming tense, which would enhance her perception of the pain. She had lost all sense of control over her headaches. Clare consumed large quantities of medication in response to her headaches, a factor that worried her husband, although she fell short of the IHS classification criteria for drug-induced headaches.

The long-term effect of decreased social and leisure activities interacted with the setting factor of no hobbies or interests.

Case II: Frank

Frank was a 37-year-old married construction programmer with two young children, referred to me by his family practitioner for headaches with an 18-year history. Frank had lived locally all his life. He completed a diploma in drafting and started studies in building, which he did not finish. He had worked as a draftsman for 16 years but had taken up a position as a construction programmer 2 years before our first appointment. Frank said that he had become fed up with being a draftsman and that his current position was a great opportunity. He enjoyed his work as a construction programmer.

Frank had been married for 15 years to Hazel, age 32. Hazel worked 2 days a week as a typist. They had two children, a son age 8 and a daughter age 3. Frank came from a large family; he had three brothers and three sisters. His parents and all his siblings lived locally but they did not spend a great deal of time together. Frank described himself as a nonpracticing Roman Catholic. He did not smoke cigarettes and drank two glasses of red wine a day.

Frank scored 21 on the BDI (long form), which placed him in the moderate depression category. His scores for the STAI placed him on the 47th percentile for state anxiety and the 42nd percentile for trait anxiety.

Frank described his headaches as a pulsating pain which occurred bilaterally behind the eyes and in the frontal region. The headaches were always preceded by sore eyes, followed approximately 1 hour later by vertigo which lasted for about an hour before the headache began. These two prodromal symptoms continued during the course of the headaches. Other symptoms associated with the headaches were photophobia and phonophobia. When the headaches were severe, they were accompanied by tremor and nausea. Frank had come close to vomiting but had never actually done so.

Frank reported that the average duration of his headaches was 4 hours. He said that they were more common in the afternoon and evening and were generally better on weekends. Self-monitoring revealed a very variable pattern, however. Inspection of the daily cards indicated that the headaches occurred daily and lasted from 1 to 14 hours. Up to three headache episodes could occur in a day. Intensity ratings ranged from 1 to 4. The headaches sometimes delayed sleep onset but did not result in waking.

Before referral, Frank had been seen by a neurologist who completed a general physical and neurological examination. The neurologist had also organized X-rays and a cranial CAT scan. None of these investigations resulted in significant findings. Frank had been assessed by several ophthalmologists who prescribed glasses which helped his vision but not his headaches. He had been treated by a physiotherapist and two acupuncturists. Only the acupuncture brought some slight relief.

Frank's family practitioner had prescribed Inderal for his headaches which Frank believed had not helped the problem. He also consumed Panadol and Codral, which brought some transitory relief, and used Vibra for his "dry" eyes. In the past he had taken a lot of Mersyndol. Self-monitoring revealed that the number of medications consumed in a day varied from two to six.

Frank's headaches fulfilled the criteria for migraine without aura. The hypothesized controlling variables of his headaches are shown in Figure 8.2. With respect to the immediate antecedents of headaches, as revealed by questioning and the change and control cards, a variety of visual stimuli would precipitate headaches, including flicker, glare, eyestrain, and looking at VDT screens. Frank's work necessitated his viewing computer screens for 2 or 3 hours at a time, and a headache tended to develop after approximately 30 minutes. He had tried alternative screens and lighting, but it had not helped. Loud noise was another perceptual stimulus that precipitated headaches, and

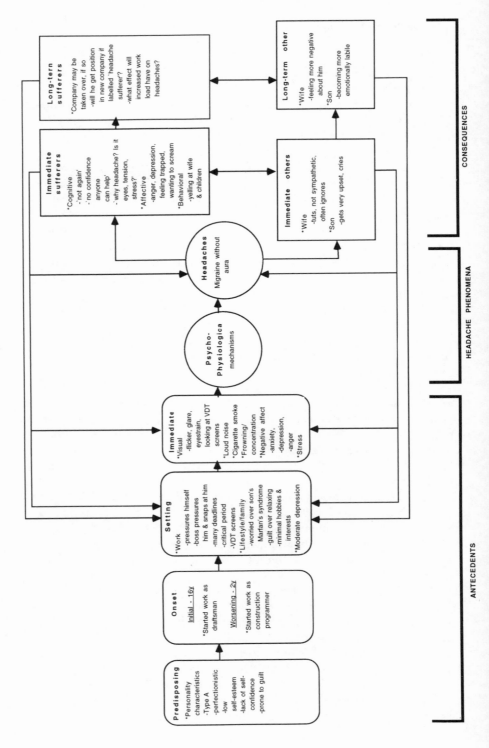

140

smoking by others could induce a headache. Headaches were also pre-cipitated and aggravated by stress, anxiety, depression, and anger.

A number of aspects of Frank's work situation seemed to serve as setting factors for his headaches. As a consequence of his perfectionistic charac-ter (predisposing factor), he consistently drove and pressured himself. His boss also had very high standards and pressured him. This man apparently watched Frank closely and snapped at him if he wasn't totally satisfied with his work. Also, the small company that Frank worked for was going through a critical period created by recessionary economic conditions and was likely to be taken over by another company, all creating additional stresses. Frank's position necessitated his spending a lot of time looking at computer screens, which led to headaches.

Other setting factors arose from Frank's domestic circumstances. His son suffered from Marfan's syndrome which is not curable and can lead to serious problems with the heart valves in the late teens. The symptoms also resulted in his son's peers making adverse comments about his appearance. Also, Frank found it very difficult to relax and enjoy himself. He felt that when he was not at work he should be helping his wife with the children or working on the house. If he wasn't engaged in these activities he felt guilty, a response that partly evolved from the fact that his wife never spent any time doing anything for herself. This guilt resulted, for example, in his never reading a newspaper but only skimming through it, unless on holiday. Although he had had many hobbies and interests in the past, including tennis, squash, sail boarding, yachting, and canoeing, at the time of referral he only played tennis once a week or every 2 weeks.

Frank's moderate depression could also be viewed as a setting factor for his headaches.

Frank's headaches had begun 18 years previously when he was age 19 and started to work as a draftsman. Over the years the headaches had become progressively more frequent, more intense, and longer in duration. The headaches became significantly worse 2 years previously, when he began his new job.

Frank was not aware of any family members or friends who suffered from regular headaches. There were a number of aspects of his personality, howev-er, that seemed likely to predispose him to developing headaches or other stress-related problems. Because Frank seemed to suffer from "hurry sick-ness," a Framingham Type A questionnaire was administered. His score was .733, which placed him in the Type A category. Frank's perfectionism combined with low self-esteem and lack of self-confidence seemed to set him up for problems at work, because he was always aspiring to high standards

←——————————————————————————————————

FIGURE 8.2. Functional model of Frank's headaches.

without believing he could, or subsequently had, achieved them. His propensity toward feeling guilty underlay his inability to take time out for recreation and relaxation.

Regarding the consequences of the headaches, Frank's cognitive responses included thoughts such as not again, and ruminations to the effect that no one could help him. He also spent time trying to analyze the headaches: Is it my eyes? Is it tension? Am I under stress? Affective responses included anger, depression, feeling trapped, and wanting to scream. When he got angry, he would shout at his wife and children.

Frank's wife and son always knew when he had a headache. Hazel's reactions included tuting (communicating disapproval) because she was so used to them. Frank believed that she tried to be sympathetic but did not succeed. Often she simply ignored his headaches. Frank's son got very distressed by his father's headaches and would become emotional and cry.

Frank claimed that his headaches had not affected his work or the family's social life. However, he spent a great deal of time worrying about the fact that the headaches might affect his work. He was concerned about the implications of his company being bought by another company. He ruminated about whether there would be a position for him in the new company if he was perceived to be a headache sufferer. He worried about whether he could cope with an increased workload in a new company in view of his headache problem. If he wasn't offered a position in the new company he envisaged his options as returning to work as a draftsman, or setting up his own business as a construction programmer. He didn't want to do the former and doubted his ability to do the latter.

The headaches affected the family in several ways. Hazel was more negatively disposed toward him because of his moods and his yelling at her and the children. Frank believed that his son had become more emotionally labile and sensitive as a result of the frequent upsets caused by the headaches.

With respect to headache mechanisms, on the antecedent side, two sets of factors stand out: stress and emotion, and visual stimuli. Words such as *worry, pressure,* and *stress* constantly arose in taking a history and appeared on the change cards prior to headaches beginning or getting worse. Frank first got headaches when he started work as a draftsman, a job that involved both visual factors (eyestrain through working on drawings) and perceived pressure arising from an interaction between the demands of the position and his personal style. The headaches got worse following a job change that exacerbated these factors. Worries over his son's syndrome and inability to find time for leisure pursuits also created a psychosocial context in which the headaches thrived. In addition to emotional and visual triggers, loud noise, cigarette smoke, and frowning could induce headaches.

Frank's responses to the headaches were maladaptive. His cognitive, affective, and behavioral responses exacerbated the stress and negative affect that precipitated the headaches, thus creating a vicious cycle. His focusing on the pain and his sense of lack of control enhanced pain perception. There was little evidence of reinforcement mechanisms operating, and although he consumed medication regularly he fell well short of the criteria for drug-induced headaches.

The longer-term effect of Frank's ruminating about the potential effect of his headaches on his career interacted with the setting factor of Work Stressors.

III

PSYCHOLOGICAL TREATMENT OF HEADACHES

"I'm very brave generally," he went on in a low voice: "only today I happen to have a headache."

—LEWIS CARROLL

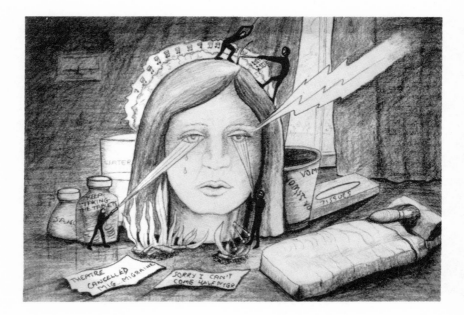

9

Planning Treatment, Parameters of Treatment, and the Educational Component

Planning a Treatment Program

The functional model of chronic headaches emphasizes that interventions can be targeted at a number of different levels. Using the terminology of the model, one level is "headache phenomena" which subdivides into the experience of headache and underlying psychophysiological mechanisms. The traditional forms of psychological treatment—biofeedback training and relaxation training—have been aimed at the psychophysiological mechanisms, while cognitive coping training has adopted a broader approach and involved other levels of the model. Although biofeedback training and relaxation training have targeted psychophysiological mechanisms, the evidence reviewed in Chapter 5 suggests that the success of these approaches derived from other effects of the treatment procedures. Holroyd's theory of how EMG biofeedback training achieves its success (Holroyd et al., 1984), for example, focused on the role of cognitive changes, such as increased feelings of self-efficacy and a more internal locus of control, and modified coping responses to headache-eliciting situations. In terms of the functional model, this theory suggests that EMG biofeedback training reduces headaches by impacting headache experience, as pain is perceived as less intense when individuals have a sense of control over their pain, and affecting stress-related immediate and setting factors.

Should treatment for headaches focus on psychophysiological mechanisms? I argue against such an orientation at present given that our understanding of the mechanisms involved is limited. As stress and negative affect appear to play a role in the development of a significant number of headaches, it seems likely that elevated arousal is a factor in such cases. It is unclear, however, precisely how this arousal manifests and leads to headaches. Also, the most promising psychophysiological data implicate vascular mechanisms which are difficult for clinicians to measure or modify. Biofeedback training is the treatment that most directly focuses on psychophysiological mechanisms, and it has not proved to be more successful than alternatives.

As future research clarifies the nature of headache mechanisms, treatment approaches that focus on them may prove to be important components of a management program. Of course, the argument against targeting psychophysiological mechanisms does not preclude the use of relaxation training. Relaxation training may alter the headache experience in a number of ways. Pain perception is adversely affected by anxiety, focusing attention on the pain, and the feeling of lack of control over the pain, as noted in Chapter 4. Relaxation training could plausibly modify any of these three factors; that is, reduce anxiety, distract from pain, or enhance feelings of self-control. Alternatively, relaxation training could affect antecedent factors such as stress, anxiety, and anger or consequences factors such as responding to headaches with negative affect. In fact, given that relaxation training is straightforward to administer and requires no special equipment, and a great deal of evidence supports its efficacy as a treatment for headaches, it is hard to see how omitting it from a headache treatment program could be justified.

Should treatment for headaches focus on the headache experience itself? There are some obvious advantages to doing so. First, the one factor shared by all headache sufferers is that they regularly experience headaches, and focus on the pain makes no assumptions about psychophysiological mechanisms or controlling variables. Also, targeting the head pain directly has high face validity for the patients. Pain management strategies have been investigated extensively in the pain literature but somewhat minimally in the headache literature. This probably reflects the fact that treatment could focus on hypothesized mechanisms for headache sufferers but not for sufferers from some other common types of pain problems such as low back pain, because the mechanisms of low back pain are not known.

All the headache treatment programs that have included a cognitive element (e.g., those of Holroyd, Blanchard, Bakal, and Martin) have included pain management strategies. Such strategies use imagery and attention techniques to modify the pain experience. Relaxation training and these other pain management techniques are discussed in Chapter 10. They tend to be appropriate for all headache sufferers.

The functional model suggests that other potential levels of intervention relate to the controlling variables of headaches (i.e., their antecedents and consequences). With respect to antecedents, one possibility is to focus on the immediate factors that precipitate or aggravate headaches. Uncontrolled studies reviewed previously by Blau and Thavapalan (1988) and Dalton (1973) have reported good treatment results simply by encouraging headache sufferers to avoid trigger factors. In some cases, this approach has considerable appeal. If an individual suffers headaches when he or she attends loud, smoky parties, there is a certain logic in suggesting that he or she participate in fewer such events. On the other hand, Philips (1987a) has argued that avoidance behavior plays a role in maintaining chronic pain because it increases sensitivity to pain-inducing stimuli. Perhaps the way to treat a headache precipitated or aggravated by visual stimuli such as glare and flicker is to "desensitize" the sufferer by exposure to these stimuli. Whether avoidance or exposure is superior is a question for future research. Clinicians meanwhile have the option of using whichever seems more appropriate in specific circumstances and changing strategies if the desired effect is not achieved.

The setting factors for headaches often provide opportunities for intervention. In the case of stress-related headaches, treatment may focus on appraisal or coping processes or increasing the perceived availability of social support. Alternatively, if stress is evolving from a particular source such as marital dysfunction or difficulties in managing children, treatment might concentrate on trying to resolve these problems.

Onset factors are less often a focus of treatment for a number of reasons. First, they are difficult to determine with any confidence because most headache sufferers do not present to psychologists until they have had headaches for many years. Second, onset factors may have no significance for the maintenance of the problem. Onset factors are included in the functional model because patients want to understand why their headaches began when they did, and because the onset factors sometimes affect the way a clinician conceptualizes the problem.

Similarly, predisposing factors are rarely a focus of treatment. They are defined as largely determined prior to birth or in the first few years of life before headache onset, so they are likely to be less amenable to change than setting and immediate factors. Nevertheless, some factors that could be categorized as predisposing might seem appropriate targets for interventions such as the Type A personality or behavioral style. Again, predisposing factors are included in the functional model because of patients' need to know why they suffer from recurrent headaches while other individuals do not, and because they contribute to the clinician's understanding of the problem.

Turning to the consequences of headaches, the immediate responses of sufferers always seem an appropriate target for intervention. Sufferers invariably respond to headaches in ways that create vicious cycles by exacerbating antecedent factors or the headache experience itself. Reactions of significant others may be an appropriate focus if, for example, reinforcement mechanisms seem to be operating, or if they respond in ways that create further stress.

The long-term effects of headaches are less likely to be a target for intervention. Long-term effects often interact with setting factors, however, so that interventions aimed at setting factors can also be aimed at long-term effects. As with predisposing and onset factors, long-term effects are included in the functional model to give patients and clinicians as broad a perspective of the headache problem as possible.

Treatment techniques focusing on the antecedents and consequences of headaches are discussed in Chapter 11.

In summary, the functional model includes 10 "boxes" any of which may suggest focuses for treatment. The factors most likely to generate treatment goals are immediate and setting antecedents, the headache experience, and the immediate reactions of sufferers. Strategies aimed at the headache experience are not likely to vary greatly from one headache sufferer to another. Stress management techniques targeted at stress-related antecedents and stress reactions to headaches are also likely to be appropriate for most headache sufferers. Other treatment techniques will vary depending on the specific controlling variables of the headaches.

Treatment Parameters and Relapse Prevention

The approach described in this book usually takes 10 to 15 50-minute sessions to complete, including assessment. Sessions are scheduled weekly while new, major techniques are being introduced and then every 2 weeks until termination.

Sessions begin with the collection of self-monitoring records and then proceed in three phases:

1. *Review.* The first phase consists of a review of what has occurred since the previous session. It starts with an open-ended question whose objective is to give patients the opportunity to tell the therapist about significant life events, fluctuations in their problems, insights that they have had, and so forth. Responses to this question may force the therapist to reconsider his or her agenda for the session. The review then focuses on self-monitoring and homework assignments, with the aim of reinforcing patients' efforts, and identifying and resolving problems that have occurred.

2. *Treatment techniques.* The second phase, which usually takes the greater part of the session, consists of using the various techniques that comprise the treatment plan. One to three techniques are used within a single session, but rarely more than one technique if it is new to the patient.

3. *Homework assignments.* The final phase involves setting up homework assignments and self-monitoring.

The treatment program concludes with a session that reviews progress and aims to maximize the chances of maintaining treatment gains. Maintenance procedures involve anticipating events and circumstances that could lead to relapse and how the patient can cope successfully with them. The patient and therapist must discuss which techniques the patient will continue to use and how he or she will use them (e.g., on a regular basis or in response to the headaches getting worse). Agreement should be reached on whether there will be any follow-up sessions and what the patient will do if his or her efforts to cope with increased headaches are unsuccessful.

Educational Component

Once assessment has been completed, a model of the patient's headaches constructed, and a treatment plan developed, management moves into the educational phase. The educational component occurs in Session 3 or 4, depending on the length of the assessment. It takes between 30 and 50 minutes to complete depending on how quick patients are to grasp the concepts and how much they wish to discuss the information presented. The educational component builds on the Preassessment Patient Information Sheet (Appendix 3) and discussions that have taken place during the preceding assessment sessions.

To understand the goals of the educational phase, it is necessary to consider the experiences and attitudes that referred patients bring with them. Most headache sufferers have had headaches for many years before they seek help from psychologists (my referrals average about 17 years). They have usually been assessed and treated by a number of medical practitioners and other health professionals, typically without gaining much relief.

What have they learned from these contacts and other experiences related to their headaches? Although health professionals vary in terms of how much information and explanation they offer, most headache sufferers seem to have learned rather little from them. The usual emphasis is on diagnosis and treatment rather than on enlightening the patient. Nevertheless, headache sufferers try to make sense of their problem, which usually results in their drawing one of two types of conclusions. Either the headaches are viewed as an inevitable consequence of their dire life circumstances, or they occur as a result of some personality defect (they are neurotic, cannot cope with stress/life, etc.). Headache sufferers often feel accused or blamed for their headaches by their doctors, families, colleagues, or friends.

As a result of the explanations sufferers construct for their headaches, and the unsuccessful treatments, they begin to feel depressed and helpless. They lose confidence in the ability of health professionals to find solutions and harbor negative expectations with respect to future treatments. Headache sufferers also develop implicit models of the treatment process. For example, health professionals are labeled "experts," and the patient's role is defined as a passive one: His or her only responsibility is to be compliant.

The goals of the educational component are to counteract these knowledge deficits, distorted beliefs, and negative attitudes that present barriers to successful psychological treatment. Outlined below is a four-stage sequence recommended for achieving these goals. Presentation of information should include handouts and can be facilitated by the use of interactive teaching aids such as white boards or overhead projectors. The educational component begins with presenting the agenda for the four-stage sequence.

Intervention Model

In the first stage, patients are told that there are three main assumptions underlying the treatment approach:

1. *Collaboration between therapist and patient.* It is assumed that both the therapist and patient have knowledge relevant to the patient's headaches. The therapist has general knowledge about headaches and how they should be assessed and treated. The patient has specific knowledge about his or her own headaches based on observations, insights, etc., over many years. The therapist's role will not be to "cure" patients but more to help them help themselves. The patient's role is an active one.

2. *Headaches arise from transactions between the patient and his or her environment, including responses to the headaches themselves.* The first phase of treatment is for the therapist and patient to achieve a mutual understanding of how the headaches arise from these transactions and to design a treatment plan accordingly. Treatment involves learning a number of skills relating to managing headache-eliciting situations and head pain and making changes to life-style.

3. *Importance of patient's efforts between office sessions.* Appointments with the therapist are only a small part of the treatment program. Patients need to collect assessment information between sessions. They also need to practice skills and to experiment with life-style changes between sessions.

The intervention model requires considerable effort on behalf of the patients.

Functional Model of Chronic Headaches

The second stage of the educational phase begins with a general discussion of headaches based on the functional model (Figure 1.1). The emphasis is on headache mechanisms and, in particular, on countering beliefs that suggest that headaches are inevitable and unchangeable. Headache phenomena are considered first. Patients are told that most people have experienced headaches and that recurrent headaches are quite common. In fact, it has been estimated that 55% of the population experience at least one mild headache per month, and 25% experience at least one mild headache each week. Further, 10% experience at least one severe headache per week, and 5% experience several severe headaches each week. These figures are derived from Nikiforow and Hokkanen (1978) and are included for two reasons: (1) to ensure that patients realize they are far from alone in their problem, and (2) to point out that a realistic goal of treatment is a reduction in headaches rather than their total elimination.

Patients are told that traditionally headaches have been divided into tension headaches and migraines, with the former caused by tense muscles around the head and the latter caused by dilated arteries in the region of the head. They are informed that recent research has case some doubt on the value of this distinction and that it will not be emphasized in their management. Likewise, they are told that research findings have questioned the role of muscle tension in headaches and so the focus will be on the role of arteries in producing pain.

With respect to antecedents, patients are told that many different factors can precipitate or aggravate headaches, including stress and negative feelings such as anxiety, anger, and depression; visual stimuli such as flicker, glare, and eyestrain; fasting, alcohol, and certain foods such as chocolate, cheese, and oranges; weather conditions such as high humidity, high temperature, and changes in weather; and hormonal factors for female sufferers such as phases of the menstrual cycle. Mechanisms by which these factors cause headaches are not entirely clear but many of these factors are known to affect the state of dilation of cranial and extracranial arteries. Patients are told that headache sufferers are sometimes not aware of the triggers of their headaches. It is suggested that headaches cannot occur "out of the blue," but trigger factors may not be obvious because of the complexities of headache mechanisms. For example, headaches may result from several factors operating together none of which individually has sufficient strength to be noticeable but which in the aggregate can induce a headache. Also, the temporal relationship between triggers and headaches (such as headaches occurring after rather than during stress) may obscure observation of the association.

Setting antecedents are introduced as the life-style or life-situation factors that make individuals vulnerable to headaches. Examples are offered, such as marital problems or difficulty managing one's children. Care must be taken when discussing setting and immediate factors not to give patients the impression that headaches are an inevitable response to certain life circumstances. Hence, it should be emphasized that it is not situations or events per se that

cause headaches but an individual's reactions (cognitive, affective, and behavioral) to the situations and events. This point is developed further when
treatment focuses on cognitive processes as mediating variables (see Chapter
11).

Onset antecedents are explained as the processes or events that resulted
in the headaches' first becoming a problem or a significantly worse problem.
Examples are given such as stressful events and hormonally mediated events
leading to headaches.

Some individuals seem to be predisposed to experiencing regular
headaches. Patients are informed that there is a slight tendency for headaches
to run in families and that there is probably a small genetic component to
headaches. They are told that predispositional factors are not well understood,
however, and are not of major etiological significance. Certain personality
characteristics may predispose individuals to developing certain types of
headaches or other disorders, but it is absolutely not the case that all headache
sufferers are in any sense neurotic, or that individuals with certain types of
personality will inevitably experience headaches.

With respect to consequences, it is emphasized to patients that the way
they respond to headaches and the way significant others react to their
headaches will affect the headache experience and the likelihood of future
headaches occurring. Examples are given such as sufferers becoming tense,
anxious, and frustrated in response to a stress-induced headache, thus creating a vicious cycle; and sufferers becoming angry with their partners, thus
provoking retaliation in the short term and marital discord in the longer term,
both of which again can result in a vicious cycle. It is important to emphasize
that becoming distressed by a severe headache is a very natural reaction but
that such a response does aggravate the problem.

I avoid providing examples of reinforcement mechanisms, except in the
case of headache sufferers for whom such mechanisms seem to be operating,
because the topic is an extremely sensitive one.

The long-term effects of headaches for both sufferers and significant
others are discussed and how these effects can play a role in an individual's
headache career. Examples are provided such as headaches leading to decreased social and recreational activities, which can aggravate setting factors
such as limited hobbies and interests, and low levels of social support.

Model of Patient's Headaches

In this stage, the controlling variables of the patient's headaches are discussed,
using a figure drawn up for the individual case, as illustrated in Figures 8.1
and 8.2. The same sequence is used as in discussing the general model:
headache phenomena (including diagnosis); immediate, setting, onset, and

predisposing antecedents; immediate reactions (sufferer and significant others) and long term effects (sufferer and significant others).

A major difference between this stage and the previous one is in the style of interaction between the therapist and patient. The general model is presented in a didactic fashion while the specific model is presented more as a series of hypotheses and propositions that are open for discussion. Patients are strongly encouraged to comment on and criticize the proposed model in order to develop a revised model that both therapist and patient think adequately represents the patient's headaches. This stage of the educational component explicitly acknowledges the patient's expertise and encourages him or her to engage with the therapist in a collaborative treatment process.

Treatment Program

The final stage of the educational component involves discussion of the proposed treatment program. Patients are told what techniques are planned to be used, including information about associated homework assignments. A brief rationale for each technique is offered including how it relates to the model of the patient's headaches discussed previously. Treatment rationales are discussed in more detail immediately prior to using the technique. Patients are given information about the proposed scheduling of techniques and how long it is estimated that treatment will take. They are invited to comment on the plan and express any concerns or reservations that they have.

The expected outcome of the program is discussed. The aim is to instill confidence without complacency and positive but not unrealistic expectations. Patients are told that they will learn some skills and make some life-style changes that should be generally useful to them. They are informed that the treatment program will almost certainly reduce their headaches, although it is impossible to predict with any degree of accuracy whether the reduction will be minimal or major.

Gate-Control Theory of Pain

Many psychological pain management programs include discussion of the gate-control theory (Melzak & Wall, 1988) in their educational component (e.g., Turk, Meichenbaum, & Genest, 1983; Philips, 1988). As the topics outlined above take some time to discuss, and coverage of the gate-control theory is not critical to the approach advocated, it is not routinely included. In some cases, however, such as when patients find it difficult to understand or accept how psychological and physical factors interact to create the pain experience, or when they are eager to discuss pain in more depth, a simplified account of the theory can be useful.

10

Focus on Headache Phenomena

Relaxation Training

As noted in Chapter 5, the main relaxation techniques used with headache sufferers are versions of progressive relaxation and autogenic training. The research literature provides little guidance as to which form of relaxation training the clinician should use with headache sufferers. Few comparisons between the different approaches have been made, although Janssen and Neutgens (1986) found that progressive relaxation was effective with tension headache and migraine sufferers but autogenic training was relatively in-effective with tension headache cases. There is certainly more research evidence supporting the efficacy of progressive relaxation than autogenic training. On the other hand, some authors report that a number of headache sufferers experience pain and discomfort on tensing muscles in the region of the head, or have difficulty releasing tension in these muscles. These writers consequently advocate forms of autogenic training for all headaches sufferers or this subgroup (Bakal, 1982; Turk et al., 1983).

I have seen such problems in only a small proportion of cases, and have found that the difficulties can be overcome by asking patients to generate less tension for shorter periods of time in the affected muscles. In view of the strong empirical support for progressive relaxation, this section focuses on this technique. Autogenic training is discussed briefly as an alternative: Certainly some patients prefer autogenic training to progressive relaxation, and the former can be practiced less obtrusively. A new approach to relaxation, namely behavioral relaxation training (BRT), is also considered briefly.

Progressive Relaxation

The original form of progressive relaxation was developed by the physiologist Edmund Jacobson (1938). The technique as proposed by Jacobson could take up to 200 hour-long sessions, reducing its clinical utility, so Wolpe (1958) introduced an abbreviated version that could be completed in six 20-minute sessions. In 1973, Bernstein and Borkovec published a 66-page manual and accompanying videotape outlining a progressive relaxation training program that took up to 10 sessions to complete. This program, with variations appropriate to chronic headache patients, is summarized below. Readers unfamiliar with this technique should study the original manual prior to using the approach.

SETTING AND RATIONALE

Relaxation training should be conducted in a setting that reduces extraneous stimuli so that the patient can concentrate on sensations of tension and relaxation. Hence, sights and sounds from outside should be reduced to a minimum, steps should be taken to avoid interruption, and lighting should be dimmed. The patient should sit in a chair that provides complete support. High-back reclining chairs are most suitable. Given the variation in size and shape between patients, it is useful to have pillows available so that the chair can be adjusted. Finally, at the session prior to beginning relaxation training, patients should be encouraged to wear comfortable, loose-fitting clothing. Patients are requested to remove items such as glasses, contact lenses, watches, rings, and shoes during relaxation training.

During the educational component of the program, as described in the previous chapter, patients were given a brief rationale for why relaxation training should help. This information is elaborated on immediately prior to commencing training. Patients are told that relaxation training has proven to be an effective treatment for headaches and a number of other problems such as anxiety and insomnia, its benefits probably derive from reducing the tension and anxiety that cause or aggravate headaches, or arise in response to head pain.

Patients are informed that the most established type of relaxation training is called progressive relaxation. Treatment will start with training in this approach but alternatives will be considered if the patient is uncomfortable with it. Progressive relaxation training involves learning to sequentially tense and then relax various groups of muscles all through the body, while paying close attention to the feelings associated with both states. The aim of progressive relaxation is to help individuals learn to recognize tension and relaxation as they occur in everyday situations. It takes several sessions to work through a training program, and the patient will need to practice at home for about 20 minutes, at least once but ideally twice each day. Patients are told that relaxation is a skill like playing tennis: For any individual to achieve his or her full potential, he or she must practice regularly. Relaxation is presented as an active coping skill that patients can use in headache-eliciting situations or to combat head pain, rather than a procedure that will automatically reduce headaches (Goldfried & Trier, 1974).

Training progresses through a number of phases and patients are briefed on each phase prior to being given relaxation instructions.

TENSION-RELEASE CYCLES

Following Bernstein and Borkovec (1973), relaxation training begins with 16 muscle groups, then combines some of these groups to form 7 groups, finally combining more groups to form 4 groups. The muscle groups are shown in Table 10.1

Bernstein and Borkovec outline a series of five events which must occur for each muscle group:

1. *The patient's attention should be focused on the muscle group.* For example, "Okay now I'd like you to focus all of your attention on the muscles of your right hand and lower arm."

2. *At a predetermined signal from the therapist, the muscle group is tensed.* For example, "All right, by making a tight fist, I'd like you to tense the muscles in the right hand and lower arm, *now.*"

3. *Tension is maintained for a period of 5 to 7 seconds* (this duration is slightly shorter for the feet as there is a danger of cramping). For example,

TABLE 10.1. Muscle Groups Involved in Progressive Relaxation Training

	Number of groups		
Muscle groups	16	7	4
Dominant hand and forearm	1	1	1
Dominant biceps	2	1	1
Nondominant hand and forearm	3	2	1
Nondominant biceps	4	2	1
Forehead	5	3	2
Upper cheeks and nose	6	3	2
Lower cheeks and jaw	7	3	2
Neck and throat	8	4	2
Chest, shoulders, and upper back	9	5	3
Abdominal or stomach region	10	5	3
Dominant thigh	11	6	4
Dominant calf	12	6	4
Dominant foot	13	6	4
Nondominant thigh	14	7	4
Nondominant calf	15	7	4
Nondominant foot	16	7	4

"Feel the muscles pull, notice what it's like to feel tension in these muscles as they pull and remain hard and tight."

4. *At a predetermined cue, the muscle group is released.* For example, "Okay *relax.*"

5. *The patient's attention is maintained upon the muscle group as it relaxes for 30 to 40 seconds.* For example, "Just let these muscles go, noticing the difference between tension and relaxation, focusing on the feeling in this muscle group as it becomes more and more relaxed."

Verbatim examples of instructions that can be used in progressive relaxation can be found in many sources in addition to the ones already cited (e.g., Blanchard & Andrasik, 1985; Wolpe & Lazarus, 1966; Goldfried & Davison, 1976). Memorizing scripts is not recommended. It can sound stilted and unnatural and also the procedure should be individualized according to the patient's level of intelligence and education.

Turk et al. (1983) make a number of points about using relaxation training with sufferers from chronic pain that are applicable to headache cases. First, particular attention should be given to muscles in the pain area (i.e., head and neck). Second, some of the earlier relaxation scripts were susceptible to disproof by, for example, telling the patient that a muscle group was relaxed when the patient might consider it otherwise. Turk et al. consequently recommend that patients should be encouraged to notice any differences taking place and to *interpret* the changes as becoming more relaxed. Finally, they emphasize that relaxation is under the patient's own control by statements such as, "Notice the changes *you* bring about."

Bernstein and Borkovec recommend that each of the muscle groups be tensed and relaxed twice. They also suggest that the therapist should determine whether deep relaxation has been achieved in one muscle group before moving on to the next. This is achieved by asking patients to raise their little finger if the relevant muscle group feels completely relaxed.

In addition to patient feedback as the session progresses, I recommend that measures of relaxation be carried out before and after administering relaxation instructions. This can be accomplished by self-report using an instrument such as the 7-point rating scale with descriptors of relaxation or arousal developed by Schilling and Poppen (1983) or observation using the Behavioral Relaxation Scale discussed subsequently.

CONCLUDING RELAXATION SESSION AND HOME PRACTICE

Relaxation instructions conclude with the therapist's counting backwards from 4 to 1 and instructing the patient to move various parts of the body at each count. For example, "On the count of 4 I'll ask you to begin to move your legs and feet," progressing to, "On the count of 1 I'll ask you to open your eyes feeling quite calm and relaxed, very pleasantly relaxed, just as if you'd had a brief nap."

After the relaxation instructions have been completed and the patient has rated his or her relaxation level, the therapist should question the patient about his or her experience during the instructions. Starting from an open-ended question such as, "Well, how was that?" therapists should proceed to specific questions to elicit any problems. These problems should be resolved and future relaxation instructions tailored to the experience reported by the patients.

Patients should be asked to practice their developing relaxation skills once or twice a day between office sessions. Providing them with audiotapes of relaxation instructions aids home practice. These tapes can sometimes be recorded during the session, but the early relaxation sessions are often too long for this purpose. The tapes should be only 15 to 20 minutes in length. To prevent patients becoming too dependent on these tapes, the tapes need to be faded out as treatment progresses.

The therapist and patient should discuss when and where the practice will be conducted and what will be said to other individuals living in the same house. The aim is to create optimal conditions similar to those operating in the therapist's office. Issues arise in home practice, however, that are unlikely to be relevant to therapists' offices. For example, it is difficult to relax under conditions of extreme cold or heat, conditions unlikely to occur in a therapist's office but which may well prevail in a patient's home. It should be emphasized that patients need to get into the spirit of home practice, that is, learning to achieve deeper and deeper levels of relaxation, rather than viewing it as a "homework assignment." They should be encouraged to find ways to help themselves become very relaxed, for example, by playing soothing background music, and incorporating these strategies into their home practice.

Patients should be required to keep records of their home relaxation practice. Minimal records include completing columns for date, start time, and finish time. Relaxation ratings before and after practice using the same scale as employed in office sessions can be very informative. Other potentially useful information includes experience during practice and difficulties encountered. These records should be discussed with patients in office sessions to resolve problems that are occurring and to reinforce the practice and recording efforts of the patient.

RELAXATION BY RECALL AND COUNTING

After successfully performing tension-release cycles with the 16 muscle groups, following by 7 groups, then 4 groups, patients begin a new phase of training. In this phase, the tension part of the cycle is eliminated and the objective is to help patients achieve a relaxed state more quickly. Relaxation by recall utilizes the four muscle groups listed in Table 10.1. For this procedure, the therapist instructs the patient to focus on any tension in a particular muscle group and then to release the tension while recalling the feelings associated with release of that tension. Patients should be encouraged to concentrate on relaxing each muscle group for 30 to 40 seconds and then signaling whether the muscle group feels completely relaxed. If the patient indicates that the muscle group is relaxed, the therapist moves onto the next group, and if deep relaxation hasn't been achieved the patient is encouraged to focus on the residual tension and to spend another 30 to 40 seconds on releasing it. Patients should be requested to use the recall procedure in home practice.

Once patients have mastered deep relaxation using the recall procedure, Bernstein and Borkovec recommend adding a counting procedure to help patients relax more deeply. The therapist counts from 1 to 10 and instructs the patient to allow the muscles to become even more deeply and completely relaxed on each count. While counting, the therapist interjects indirect relaxation instructions, for example, "1, 2, noticing the arm and hands becoming more and more relaxed now; 3, 4, focusing on the muscles of the face and neck as they become even more deeply relaxed now," and so forth. Patients should be requested to use the counting procedure at the conclusion of recall practice at home.

Once patients have successfully integrated the recall and counting procedure into home practice, therapists can introduce a procedure which consists solely of counting from 1 to 10 and giving indirect suggestions of relaxation. If at the end of the counting procedure the patient indicates that some tension remains, the therapist should locate the residual tension and have the patient remove it through the recall technique, or if that fails through tension-release cycles. The aim of the counting procedure is to enable patients to achieve deep relaxation in the minute or less that it takes to count from 1 to 10.

CUE-CONTROLLED AND DIFFERENTIAL RELAXATION

Cue-controlled relaxation, referred to as conditioned relaxation by Bernstein and Borkovec, takes the relaxation process one stage further by associating relaxation with a cue word such as *calm* or *relax* rather than with counting. Patients achieve cue-controlled relaxation by using the previously discussed procedures and then focusing attention on breathing and subvocalizing a cue word each time they exhale. The therapist repeats the word in synchrony with exhalation five times, and the patient continues for 15 more pairings.

This procedure is practiced until the cue word can elicit the relaxation response.

Differential relaxation is based on the supposition that a variety of muscles become tensed during most behaviors, but muscles necessary for the accomplishment of an activity are frequently more tense than they need to be, and muscles unnecessary for efficient performance become tense during the activity. Differential relaxation involves inducing deep relaxation in muscles not required for an ongoing activity and eliminating excess tension in muscles involved in the activity. This is achieved by periodically identifying tension during daily activities and then relaxing muscles that are unnecessarily tense. Differential relaxation is initially practiced in relatively undemanding situations. Level of demand is defined according to three dimensions: situations (varying from being alone in a quiet room to being with others in a noisy place), position (varying from sitting to standing), and activity level (varying from inactivity to routine complex movements).

SCHEDULE FOR RELAXATION TRAINING AND PROBLEMS ENCOUNTERED

Bernstein and Borkovec suggest a 10-session timetable that includes three sessions on 16 muscle groups, two sessions on 7 groups, two sessions on 4 groups, and one session each on relaxation by recall, relaxation by recall and counting, and relaxation by counting. Differential relaxation is practiced over a 3-week period in the latter half of the program and cue-controlled relaxation at the end of the program. The first session of relaxation training tends to take the whole office session (i.e., approximately 50 minutes) because it involves 16 muscle groups and includes the treatment rationale and instructions in home practice. Subsequent relaxation sessions steadily decrease in length to periods of 10 to 15 minutes.

While Bernstein and Borkovec (1973) offer these guidelines, they repeatedly emphasize that progress both within sessions and between sessions should be determined by patient response rather than following a set timetable. New procedures are introduced after the patient has mastered the previous one. They suggest that the 10-session timetable is a conservative one and that most patients proceed more rapidly. I usually use 6 to 10 relaxation sessions with headache patients. Most of these sessions allow time for using other techniques also.

In their manual, Bernstein and Borkovec (1973) list 15 problems that can occur with relaxation training: (1) muscle cramps, (2) movement (e.g., fidgeting, scratching, stretching), (3) laughter or talking, (4) external noise, (5) spasms and tics, (6) intrusive thoughts, (7) sleep, (8) coughing and sneezing, (9) inability to relax specific muscle groups, (10) strange or unfamiliar feelings during relaxation, (11) "losing control" during relaxation, (12) "internal arousal," (13) failure to follow instructions, (14) problems with practicing, and (15) words and phrases to avoid. A problem that has been discussed more recently is "relaxation-induced anxiety" (Heide & Borkovec, 1983, 1984), or "relaxation-training-induced arousal" as Poppen (1988) has more appropriately called it. These problems are not pursued here because each occurs somewhat infrequently, most experienced clinicians would feel comfortable handling them if they did arise, and solutions have been discussed in the sources cited.

A few comments must be made, however, about patients failing to complete home relaxation practice. Headache patients vary considerably in their reaction to relaxation training and in particular to the requirement to practice developing skills between office sessions. At one extreme, some patients are delighted to be "given permission" to spend 30 to 40 minutes each day taking time out to relax; at the other extreme some patients find the practice intensely boring and a frustrating obstacle to getting on with their life. It is difficult to convince some patients to practice, while others have to be discouraged from practicing for considerably longer than requested.

Of course, such difficulties have to be resolved, but they should also be viewed as an opportunity to learn more about the patient and his or her headaches. A common pattern, for example, is for patients to practice inconsistently, which they justify on the grounds that sometimes they are too busy. This raises an interesting question: Are the headaches better or worse when patients are busier (and not practicing relaxation)? Headache and relaxation records provide a good opportunity for studying such relationships. Occasionally, the headaches diminish, which may indicate that they are more of a problem when patients have time to ruminate about them than when patients are otherwise occupied and distracted. More commonly, the headaches are worse when the patient is busy. This can be a valuable lesson to the patient, and the therapist can point out that just when patients find relaxation practice most difficult to fit into their schedule is when it is most important for them to do so.

Autogenic Training

Autogenic training was devised by the psychiatrist Johannes Schultz in the early 20th century, and following early publications in German, it was subsequently described in English (Schultz & Luthe, 1959, 1969). Schultz concentrated on the potential of autosuggestion with the aim of developing an effective psychotherapeutic approach without the negative aspects of hypnotherapy such as the passivity of the patient and his or her dependence on the therapist. Autogenic training is described by its authors as a psychophysiological approach based on the assumption that psychological and physiological processes are inexorably linked. This method seeks to regulate mental and somatic functions simultaneously by "passive concentration" on formulae such as "my forehead is cool."

Schultz and Luthe suggest that afferent stimuli must be reduced to the lowest possible physiological level during autogenic training, and they recommend settings similar to progressive relaxation. They propose three alternative training postures: lying down (the easiest), sitting in a high-back reclining chair, and sitting on a straight chair (the most frequently adopted).

Schultz and Luthe emphasize the need for passive concentration during autogenic exercises. They differentiate passive concentration from what is usually called concentration, but which they refer to as "active concentration," as follows: "Passive concentration implies a casual attitude and functional passivity toward the intended outcome of his concentrative activity, while active concentration is characterized by the person's concern, interest, attention and goal-directed active efforts during the performance of a task and in respect to the final functional result" (Schultz & Luthe, 1959, p. 10).

Schultz and Luthe describe six standard exercises, seven meditative exercises, and two special exercises. They suggest that the standard exercises take 13 to 30 weeks to complete successfully. The autogenic training program of Janssen and Neutgens (1986), which was found to be effective with migraine and combined headache sufferers, used the six standard exercises of Schultz and Luthe. In a 12-session program, each exercise was practiced for two sessions and patients were required to practice at home between sessions twice a day.

STANDARD EXERCISES

The particular form, content, and sequence of the standard formulae are based on clinical and experimental observations of psychophysiological changes that occur during sleep and hypnosis. Patients are asked to visualize the relevant part of the body and then concentrate on the corresponding autogenic formula. Patients can utilize a verbal, visual, or acoustic form of the formula.

In autogenic training, the therapist introduces each new formula. After the patient has assumed one of the three body postures and closed his or her eyes, the therapist starts repeating the formula in a low voice for about 30 to 40 seconds. A subsequent period of about 30 seconds of silence allows the patient to continue with passive concentration on the new formula. After this period, the patient comes back to normal by flexing arms and legs vigorously, breathing deeply, and opening eyes. Usually, three exercises are done successively with about 1 minute between them, during which patients are encouraged to maintain some degree of motor activity and to report on their experience during the exercise.

1. *Heaviness*. The first standard exercise is aimed at muscle relaxation. The heaviness exercise begins with the dominant arm, using the formula "my right arm is heavy" (for right-handed patients). Successive formulae focus on the nondominant arm, both arms, dominant leg, nondominant leg, both legs, and arms and legs. Schultz and Luthe suggest that passive concentration is facilitated and the physiological effect of the autogenic exercises enhanced if the first formula is associated with peaceful images that provide a calming background for the patient's state of mind. They recommend accompanying the first physiologically oriented formula of each exercise with a background formula such as "I am at peace."

2. *Warmth*. This exercise is aimed at vasodilation. During this phase of training, formulae such as "my right arm is warm" are added to the formulae already used pertaining to heaviness and peace. The sequence of limbs used for the warmth formulae are the same as for the heaviness formulae. As soon as patients can establish warmth regularly in the extremities, synoptic formulae are used such as "my arms and legs are warm."

3. *Cardiac regulation*. The third exercise aims at amplifying the psychophysiological effects of the heaviness and warmth formulae by focusing directly on the activity of the heart. The standard formula is "heartbeat calm and regular" and is interjected among already used formulae. Initially for this exercise, patients should be on their back with their right hand over their heart.

4. *Respiration*. This exercise uses the formula "my breathing is calm" or "it breathes me."

5. *Abdominal warmth*. The fifth exercise seeks to establish warmth in the depth of the abdominal cavity by focusing on the solar plexus and uses the formula "my solar plexus is warm." Since the expression *solar plexus* is unfamiliar to many·patients, explanations and pictorial demonstrations are usually required. Having patients place their hands over their abdomen is helpful for this exercise.

6. *Cooling of the forehead*. The standard training formula for the final exercise is "my forehead is cool." Schultz and Luthe warn, however, that headache patients should begin with the modified formula "my forehead is slightly cool" applied for brief periods only (20 to 30 seconds), as they have observed some headaches to get worse with this exercise. If this formula leads to an increase in pain, the alternative formula "flowing warmth in nape and shoulders" should be practiced. If the "slightly cool" formula is beneficial, the standard formula should be employed.

Behavioral Relaxation Training

In contrast to the two relaxation techniques discussed so far, BRT is a recent innovation (Poppen, 1988). BRT represents a behavior-analytic approach to relaxation training and emphasizes overt motoric behavior (Schilling & Poppen, 1983). This emphasis allows observation of progress by both the therapist and patient.

Poppen (1988) stresses that researchers and clinicians using relaxation training seldom measure what their trainees are doing and how it relates to treatment outcome. In contrast, his approach is oriented around assessment. Before discussing his training procedures, it is necessary to describe the interesting measure of relaxation that he has developed.

BEHAVIORAL RELAXATION SCALE

The basic premise of the Behavioral Relaxation Scale (BRS) is that a relaxed person engages in overt motor behavior that is characteristic of relaxation, and it is possible for an observer to judge how relaxed an individual is from these behaviors. The BRS consists of a description of 10 postures and activities characteristic of a relaxed person whose body is fully supported by a reclining chair. The 10 relaxed behaviors pertain to head, eyes, mouth, throat, shoulders, body, hands, feet, quiet (no vocalization or loud respiratory sounds), and breathing. For each item on the BRS, the relaxed behavior and the corresponding unrelaxed behavior are described. Pictures accompany the descriptions. To use eyes as an example, relaxed consists of "the eyelids are lightly closed with a smoother appearance and no motion of the eyelids" (p. 30), and unrelaxed consists of "(a) Eyes open. (b) Eyelids closed but wrinkled or fluttering. (c) Eyes moving under the lids" (p. 30).

Using the BRS requires an observation period of 5 minutes. Each minute of this period is divided into three intervals: 30 seconds to observe breathing rate, 15 seconds to observe the other nine relaxation behaviors, and 15 seconds for recording the observations on a score sheet. The BRS score for each observation period is a percentage based on the number of behaviors scored as relaxed or unrelaxed, divided by the total number of observations.

The procedural validity of the BRS has been demonstrated by showing that relaxation procedures (EMG biofeedback training, progressive relaxation, and BRT) produced significant changes on the BRS while a credible placebo procedure did not (Schilling & Poppen, 1983). Also, the concurrent validity has been established by showing that relaxed and unrelaxed behaviors, as defined by the BRS, were related to tension levels in relevant muscle groups (Poppen & Maurer, 1982).

TRAINING PROCEDURES

BRT proceeds by teaching individuals to "look relaxed." The typical BRT session involves the following phases: (1) adaptation (5–10 minutes), (2) pretraining observation (5 minutes), (3) acquisition (first session only) (15–30 minutes), (4) proficiency training (15–30 minutes), and (5) posttraining observation (5 minutes).

Acquisition involves four steps for each of the 10 behaviors listed in the BRS. First, each behavior is given a one-word label by which it can be conveniently identified (e.g., hands, feet). Second, the relaxed behavior is described and demonstrated by the therapist; commonly occurring unrelaxed behaviors are also demonstrated. Third, the patient is asked to demonstrate the relaxed posture. Finally, the patient is given feedback. Praise is provided for correct imitation and corrective instructions otherwise. Manual guidance is employed if the patient is still unsuccessful after two or three attempts.

As each behavior is successfully imitated, the patient is asked to maintain the posture or activity for 30 to 60 seconds and to observe the feelings that occur. Patients are asked to maintain the trained behaviors as each new one is added.

After all 10 items have been learned in acquisition training, additional training is needed to reach criterion on the BRS and to promote relaxed behaviors in other response domains. Proficiency training involves instructions, systematic observation of relaxed and unrelaxed behaviors, and verbal feedback. Instructions consist of asking patients to relax all 10 areas and to review the 10 items to observe the feelings in each area. Patients are told that the therapist will observe the relaxed and unrelaxed behavior and will periodically provide feedback. Observation occurs over a 2-minute interval and the therapist provides feedback by reporting aloud the one-word label for any item noted to be unrelaxed during this period. If the label is not sufficient to prompt the patient to correct an unrelaxed area, corrective feedback can be employed.

Poppen describes three variations to BRT that enable the patient to engage in relaxed behaviors throughout the day in situations that do not allow the person to recline and totally relax. Given that reclining chairs are not commonly available in most environments, the first variation is to teach the patient to relax in an upright chair. The Upright Relaxation Scale has been derived defining postures requiring the least muscle tension to sustain while seated in an upright position. Poppen refers to the second variation as "mini-relaxation." This involves relaxing parts of the body while engaged in other activities and hence is a concept similar to differential relaxation. The final variation is diaphragmatic breathing.

As do other forms of relaxation training, BRT involves 20 minutes of home practice each day.

BRT has not yet been used in controlled trials with headache sufferers, but Poppen provides a detailed description of the successful treatment of a migraineur with his procedures. He also points out that BRT can readily be combined with other treatment procedures, including alternative relaxation techniques such as progressive relaxation and autogenic training.

Cognitive Methods: Imagery and Attention

A laboratory and clinical research literature has developed over the last two decades on the use of cognitive strategies to ameliorate pain. These strategies have been classified by Fernandez (1986) into three main categories: imagery, self-statements, and attention–diversion. This section discusses imagery and attention–diversion strategies, as these techniques focus on headache phenomena (i.e., pain management strategies) while self-statement approaches will be considered in the first section of Chapter 11, as these techniques focus on the antecedents and consequences of headaches.

Before discussing these techniques, it should be emphasized that the research literature again provides limited guidance with respect to which specific techniques to use. Controlled studies of experimental pain have produced mixed results—56% demonstrate cognitive strategies to be superior to control procedures and the remainder find no significant differences (Tan, 1982). No conclusive findings about which type of cognitive strategy is most effective have emerged from these experimental studies, although there is some evidence that strategies relevant to the sensations that are being experienced (e.g., imaginative transformation) are more effective than irrelevant strategies (e.g., imaginative inattention) that attempt to deny the existence of the sensations (Spanos, Horton, & Chaves, 1975). It is commonly suggested by reviewers that the null findings that have occurred in some studies arise because a number of experimental subjects are being instructed to use strategies that make little sense to them, and that may not be as effective as the ones that they have developed themselves during previous experience of pain. Control subjects tend to use their own cognitive strategies spontaneously (e.g., Weisenberg, 1989; Pearce, 1983).

Cognitive strategies have, of course, been employed in all the studies of cognitive therapy for chronic headache reviewed in Chapter 5, but the specific contribution of the strategies to the overall treatment package has not been determined. A study by Rybstein-Blinchik (1979) showed the superiority of a cognitive strategy involving the reinterpretation of pain compared to the strategy of diverting attention from pain for reducing the chronic pain experience. Similarly, studies by Keefe and Dolan (1986) and Turner and Clancy (1986) found that with chronic pain patients, attention–diversion strategies were associated with poorer treatment outcome.

Given the current state of the research literature, it seems appropriate to offer patients a variety of cognitive strategies and to encourage them to use the ones that make the most sense to them. Building on existing cognitive strategies and tailoring strategies to the needs of the individual are recommended (Turk et al., 1983; Hanson & Gerber, 1990). The importance of individual differences in this area was emphasized in a recent study by Heyneman, Fremouw, Gano, Kirkland, and Heiden (1990) which demonstrated that a self-statement approach was more effective than an attention–diversion approach in attenuating acute pain for subjects classified as "catastrophizers," but the reverse was the case for subjects classified as "noncatastrophizers."

Imagery Training

In Fernandez's (1986) classification of cognitive coping approaches, imagery strategies are split into the two subcategories of incompatible imagery and transformative imagery. The former refers to images of events inconsistent with pain, and subdivides into incompatible emotive imagery and incompatible sensory imagery. The aim of incompatible emotive imagery is to elicit emotions that inhibit pain. Emotions recommended for such imagery include mirth, humor, pride, and self-assertion. Incompatible sensory imagery (also known as imaginative inattention) employs images of "pure" visual, auditory, or other sensations incompatible with pain. Clinically, this imagery usually assumes the form of pleasant images of blue skies, grassy meadows, white sandy beaches, streams, and waterfalls.

Transformative imagery is designed to alter specific features of the pain experience and is subdivided into the three variations of contextual, stimulus, and response. In contextual transformation, the context or setting of the pain is altered in imagination. An often quoted example from laboratory research is of individuals who are administered forearm ischemic pain imagining themselves as spies shot in the arm and escaping from enemy agents. This colorful illustration clarifies the nature of the strategy but is unlikely to be useful with chronic headache sufferers. Imaging head pain as resulting from intense concentration on successfully solving important problems would be an example of contextual transformation.

Stimulus transformation involves the imaginative transformation of the stimulus features of the pain. For example, if head pain is experienced as a tight band around the head, this approach to imagery might involve loosening the band. Response transformation involves the imaginative transformation (or relabeling) of the pain experience without reference to the concept of pain. For example, headaches may be relabeled as feelings of pressure, tightness, or throbbing.

RATIONALE AND INITIAL PROCEDURE

Imagery training begins with a simplified account of the nature of imagery. Hence, patients are told that imagery consists of "pictures in the mind" of objects, events, and situations in the absence of the actual objects, events, or situations. It is explained that imagery represents one level of human functioning of which others are thoughts, feelings, behaviors, and physiology. Patients are told that these levels are not independent but interact with each other. For example, if an individual who is about to get on a plane develops images of a horrendous plane crash, his or her thoughts (e.g., should I take this flight?), feelings (e.g., anxiety), behavior (e.g., leaving the airport), and physiology (e.g., increased heart rate and sweating) are likely to be affected.

It is then explained to patients that because imagery is largely under voluntary control, it can be used for producing desirable changes in feelings and physiology, including counteracting headaches. In fact, most people do employ this strategy in certain stressful situations. For example, many individuals when faced with an aversive medical procedure such as an injection will cope with the event by imagining that they are engaged in their hobby or are in a favorite location, so as to distract themselves and help themselves relax.

Patients are told that individuals vary in their ability to use imagery and it can be thought of as a skill. Some individuals can produce very vivid images so that the pictures in their minds are as real as if the subject of the image was actually there in front of them; some individuals can become absorbed in their images and control them. Other individuals are lower in their imagery ability and can only produce weak images from which they are easily distracted. As with relaxation, however, the way to develop imagery skills is to practice using them. Patients are then shown scales for measuring imagery vividness and imagery control.

At this point, it is helpful to demonstrate to patients that imagery can affect the way they feel and their physiological reactions. A commonly used exercise is to encourage patients to imagine cutting a lemon and touching their tongues with a segment of it (e.g., Bakal, 1982; Turk et al., 1983). This exercise is aimed at inducing reactions such as salivation and swallowing. I have found that some patients experience minimal responses to this exercise, and I prefer to use food for the imaginal stimulus. Patients are asked what food they would most like to eat right now and are then directed to develop an image of that food. The therapist should guide the patient's efforts by describing the food in as much detail as possible. All five senses (visual, auditory, tactile, olfactory, and gustatory) should be involved in imagery training whenever appropriate. The aim is for the patient to conjure up an image that is as vivid and real as possible. If this approach doesn't produce readily detectable physiological responses (i.e., salivation), "gruesome" imagery such as visualizing scratching fingernails across a blackboard or even running fingers along a sharp knife edge usually results in reactions (i.e., shivers and shudders).

It is also useful to have the patient visualize a pleasant image. Such an image usually has less obvious physiological effects than the ones discussed above, but emphasizes to patients the positive effects that imagery can achieve. Also, this exercise serves as practice for using incompatible sensory imagery as a pain coping strategy.

After each imagery exercise, the therapist should discuss with the patient his or her experience. Patients should also be requested to rate the vividness and control of the image they produced on the scales shown to them previously.

At this point, patients are questioned about whether their headaches are associated with imagery and whether they use imagery to counteract their headaches or any other stressful situations. This is followed by a discussion of the five imagery strategies listed in the previous section. Patients who respond that they do not employ imagery often realize that they do when the five strategies are brought to their attention. For each of the imagery techniques, examples need to be developed that are personally meaningful to the patient.

HOME PRACTICE AND SUBSEQUENT PROCEDURES

Home practice for imagery training is divided into two phases: developing imagery ability and using imagery coping strategies. In the first phase, patients are encouraged to spend 10 minutes each day controlling their imagery in order to learn to develop more vivid images and to gain greater control of their imagery. A good starting point for home practice is the images used in the office session. Patients should keep records of their home practice using a format similar to the relaxation practice diaries. Hence, appropriate column headings are date, start time, finish time, and ratings of vividness of image and control of image.

Also, during the first phase of home practice, it is useful for patients to observe whether any imagery is associated with their headaches. Such imagery can be recorded in a sixth column of the practice diaries.

Once patients can reliably produce images that are reasonably vivid and controlled, the second phase of home practice can begin. This phase involves employing coping strategies to control headaches and necessitates the use of a more complex type of recording system. The system that I recommend begins with five rows labeled according to the five imagery strategies. This serves as a prompt to the patient as well as facilitating recording. Column headings can then include the ones already used (date, start time, finish time, and ratings of vividness of image and control of image), and in addition, pain intensity ratings for before and after using the imagery coping strategy.

Office sessions are used mainly to review home practice with the aid of the records. Additional imagery exercises can be helpful if patients are experiencing difficulties in producing appropriate images. A set of guidelines for the use of imagery in the management of pain has been prepared by McCaffery (1979).

Attention–Diversion Training

Attention–diversion strategies are divided into passive versus active distraction in the classification of Fernandez (1986), depending on the degree of involvement of the individual in the distractor stimulus or task. I prefer, however, to use the internal versus external dichotomy which appeared in the earlier classification of cognitive coping strategies for pain management developed by Turk (e.g., Turk & Genest, 1979).

Internal attention–diversion can be further subdivided into focusing on mental activity versus bodily processes and sensations. The former, which has been investigated more widely, involves strategies such as mental arithmetic (e.g., serial subtraction), reciting poetry, recalling the words of popular songs, and making lists of tasks to be done over the weekend. The latter involves directing attention away from headaches to bodily processes that are not associated with pain, such as breathing, or to parts of the body that are comfortable and relaxed.

External attention–diversion can be subdivided into focusing on features of the environment versus becoming involved in tasks that distract from the pain experience. The former, which has been investigated more widely, involves strategies such as the following: counting ceiling or floor tiles; studying the construction of objects present in the room; studying the shapes of clouds, trees, and houses; and detecting and analyzing sounds present in the environment. The latter consists of becoming involved in tasks or activities that distract from pain. These activities need to be sufficiently low in demand that individuals can engage in them while suffering from a headache, but sufficiently high in demand to recruit attentional resources.

RATIONALE AND INITIAL PROCEDURE

Attention–diversion training follows a similar sequence to imagery training. It begins with a discussion of attention based on Bakal (1982). Patients are told that attention has three properties relevant to using attentional processes to attenuate headaches:

1. Attentional capacity is limited so that individuals tend to focus on one thing at a time.

2. Attention is under voluntary control so that individuals can decide on what they wish to focus.

3. It is difficult if not impossible to stop paying attention to unpleasant sensations unless one refocuses on other things.

A useful analogy for communicating the first two properties to patients is to compare attention with a searchlight. Objects in the direct glare of the searchlight can be seen clearly, but those outside the beam cannot (property 1). A searchlight can be moved from focusing on one object to focusing on another (property 2).

The significance of attentional processes to headaches is explained to patients as follows: It is pointed out to them that most people are aware that pain feels worse when attention is devoted to it than when the sufferer is distracted from the pain. Everyday examples of this phenomenon are boxers and football players who sustain severe injuries during the excitement of competitive sport without being aware of the injuries until the contest is over. Hence, it is argued that attentional mechanisms can be used to attenuate headaches by refocusing attention away from the pain. Following through the searchlight analogy, the aim of attention–diversion training is to point the searchlight in a direction other than the headache, so that the pain sensations go out of focus and recede into the background.

Patients are told that the skill of using attention to ameliorate pain is in being able to control attention. Put another way, it is about the ability to concentrate and not allow oneself to be distracted by pain sensations. Attentional skills, like other skills, can be enhanced by practice. Patients are shown a scale for measuring attentional control.

At this point, an attentional exercise is carried out to demonstrate the three properties of attention discussed previously. Initially, patients are asked simply to observe where their attention is focused. Then they are requested to practice controlling their attention by focusing on internal stimuli (e.g., sensation of breathing) or external stimuli (e.g., sounds and noises) and then redirecting their attention elsewhere. Patients are asked to notice how whatever they pay attention to is clear while other objects and events tend to fade from awareness. They are also requested to stop focusing on the current object of attention and compare this with refocusing on something else, observing how much easier it is to reduce awareness of an object via the latter strategy. Following the exercise, patients are asked about their experience with it and requested to rate the degree of attentional control that they achieved during the exercise.

Patients are then asked whether they have used distraction to cope with their headaches or any other unpleasant or stressful situations. This is followed by going through the four variations of attention–diversion strategies that can be used to combat headaches. Again, the emphasis is on the therapist's working with the patient to find examples of these approaches that make the most sense to the patient. A good illustration of this individual tailoring was provided by Turk et al. (1983). These authors refer to the case of a classical musician for whom listening to a popular song was only one third as effective in increasing his pain threshold as listening to a Bach fugue.

HOME PRACTICE AND SUBSEQUENT PROCEDURES

Home practice for attention–diversion training proceeds as for imagery training. Hence, it is divided into two phases: developing control of attention and using attention–diversion strategies to control pain. During the first phase, patients are encouraged to spend 10 minutes each day directing and redirecting their attention as they did during the office session. Home practice is recorded on diaries as for imagery training. The only difference is in the rating scale used.

Once patients have had some success controlling their attention, they are requested to practice using the four types of attention–diversion strategies for attenuating pain. Records are kept as for imagery strategies.

Office sessions are used for reviewing home practice and additional attentional exercises, if warranted.

11

Focus on Antecedents and Consequences of Headaches

This chapter is structured according to the different categories of headache antecedents and consequences. It begins, however, with a section on cognitive methods that target stress- and headache-related thoughts and underlying beliefs or assumptions. These methods cut across a number of functional categories. Hence, stress-related thoughts pertain to immediate antecedents and headache-related thoughts to immediate reactions of the sufferer. The formation and activation of underlying maladaptive beliefs may be related to predisposing, onset, or setting antecedent factors.

Cognitive Methods: Thoughts and Beliefs

Rationale

The rationale for a cognitive approach focusing on maladaptive thoughts and beliefs takes 20 to 40 minutes to explain. As well as preparing the patient to target maladaptive thoughts and underlying beliefs, this rationale prepares the patient for other interventions aimed, for example, at increasing social support or decreasing anxiety and depression. The rationale proceeds in three phases; the key points are described below.

RELATIONSHIP BETWEEN HEADACHES, STRESS,
AND NEGATIVE EMOTIONS

The most common triggers of headaches are stress and negative emotions or feelings, such as anxiety, depression, and anger. It is pointed out that stress and negative feelings are difficult to disentangle because negative emotions are part of the stress response. Patients are also told that because headaches are aversive experiences they can be viewed as stressors, and indeed headaches give rise to negative emotions. This creates a vicious cycle whereby stress and negative emotions precipitate headaches, which are perceived as stressful, and in turn give rise to further negative feelings, thus completing a loop.

The implication of the stress–headache–stress cycle is that headaches can be treated by reducing the stress response and negative emotions that trigger the headaches or by making the headache experience less stressful and characterized by negative feelings, thus breaking the cycle. Patients are then told that to understand how this can be achieved, the nature of stress and emotions must first be considered.

NATURE OF STRESS AND EMOTIONS

Patients are presented with a transactional model of stress in which it is suggested that stress responses arise from an imbalance between perceived environmental demands on the one hand and perceived personal and social resources of the individual on the other (Lazarus & Folkman, 1984; Steptoe, 1991). It is explained that stress usually arises from demands exceeding resources, but the reverse can occur, particularly in monotonous working conditions where people are unable to fully utilize their skills (Theorell, 1989).

The essential features of this model are communicated to the patient by contrasting the model with popular, simplistic conceptualizations of stress. Patients are told that most people think of stress as a property of certain events or life situations. For example, examinations, divorce, or losing a job are viewed as stressful events. In fact, individuals vary considerably in the degree to which they find the same event stressful, because the stress response is mediated by the way individuals *think* about the event. In the terminology of the model, some individuals perceive the demands of exams as higher than others; that is, some individuals see exams as more threatening or taxing than do others. Of course, some extreme environmental conditions such as military combat, natural disasters, and imprisonment are generally appraised as so high in demand that they are likely to result in stress for most people. There are individual differences in reactions even to such noxious events, however, and a much greater variability in response to everyday life stressors or hassles.

An important characteristic of the model is the inclusion of perceived psychosocial resources. This latter term refers to the way an individual *thinks* about his or her ability to cope with stress personally or with the help of others (family, friends, colleagues, etc.). Situations perceived as high demand are not experienced as stressful if an individual believes that he or she has the skills or support to cope successfully with the situation. For example, whether exams are experienced as stressful depends on whether individuals see themselves as having the necessary personal resources (e.g., knowledge and ability) and social resources (e.g., support from family and friends) to meet the demands (e.g., performance required to achieve desired outcome).

In the transactional model, stress can be reduced by modifying either perceived environmental demands or perceived psychosocial resources. This can be accomplished by changing actual demands or resources (assuming perceptions change accordingly), or changing the way individuals *think* about demands (e.g., appraise event as less threatening) or resources (e.g., view oneself as more able to cope and in control).

Just as thinking is a critical intermediate factor in determining the stress response, so it is central to understanding emotions generally. The way we feel is dependent on the way we think. If, for example, an individual approaches forthcoming air travel with thoughts such as the "plane may crash," and "I might become so afraid that I will faint or vomit," he or she will experience negative emotions such as fear and anxiety. In contrast, if an individual approaches the flight with thoughts such as "I am looking forward to the flight," he or she will experience positive emotions such as relaxation and pleasure.

RELATIONSHIP BETWEEN THOUGHTS AND BELIEFS

The thoughts that play a role in the stress response and negative emotions reflect underlying beliefs or assumptions. Thoughts tend to be specific to particular situations, but assumptions are general rules that apply across situations. For example, the thought "I have let down my company by losing that contract" may be based on the underlying assumption "I must never make a mistake"; the thought "as I don't get on with Joe, I will never be a successful member of the team" may be based on the underlying assumption "I must be liked by everyone."

Finally, in view of the above, the way to change the stress responses and negative emotions that both cause and arise from patients' headaches is to modify the mediating thoughts and underlying beliefs. This is not a simple task, but it can be accomplished with training and practice.

Targets for Change

The goals of this approach are to modify maladaptive thoughts and underlying beliefs as they pertain to the three interrelated situations of stress, negative emotions, and headaches and related factors (e.g., associated symptoms and medication consumption).

STRESS-RELATED THOUGHTS

Assuming that stress is arising from perceived environmental demands exceeding perceived psychosocial resources, the aim is to modify thoughts and beliefs so as to reduce demands and increase resources. Changing perceived demands via a cognitive approach involves modifying appraisal processes so that patients view stressors as less threatening, dangerous, taxing, overwhelming, and so forth. A cognitive approach to perceived resources involves increasing patients' beliefs in their ability to control and cope with stressors.

THOUGHTS AND NEGATIVE EMOTIONS

Beck and his colleagues have listed the logical errors in thinking that are associated with depression and anxiety (e.g., Beck et al., 1979; Beck & Emery, 1985). They consist of the following:

1. *Arbitrary inference.* This involves jumping to conclusions on the basis of inadequate evidence. For example, a person who doesn't do well on one college exam assumes that he will not receive his degree (depression-type error).

2. *Selective abstraction.* This involves attending only to depressing or threatening experiences. For example, a person who is going to a dance focuses only on the potential embarrassment of no one asking her to dance (anxiety-type error).

3. *Overgeneralization.* This involves making sweeping judgments on the basis of a single experience or instance. For example, a person whose job is eliminated because of budgetary cuts concludes that he is worthless (depression-type error).

4. *Dichotomous reasoning.* This involves thinking in extremes so that all experiences are placed in one of two opposite categories. For example, situations are either unmistakably safe or unsafe, so the rustling of venetian blinds would be interpreted as indicating an intruder (anxiety-type error).

5. *Personalization.* This involves taking responsibility for things that have little or nothing to do with oneself. For example, a person blames herself for a neighbor's slipping on his path, because she believes that she should have warned the neighbor (depression-type error).

6. *Catastrophizing.* This involves dwelling on the worst possible outcome of any situation in which there is a possibility for an unpleasant outcome. For example, a person who is about to fly on a plane dwells on the possibility of the plane's crashing (anxiety-type error).

7. *Magnification and minimization.* This involves exaggerating (magnifying) limitations and difficulties while playing down (minimizing)

accomplishments, achievements, and capabilities. For example, a person reviewing his work record focuses on his failures and overlooks his successes (depression-type error).

THOUGHTS RELATED TO HEADACHES AND ASSOCIATED FACTORS

Many of the cognitive reactions to headaches and associated factors, such as accompanying symptoms and taking medication, reflect headaches as stressors and their association with negative affect. For example, a common maladaptive response to headaches is to exaggerate the demands of the situation (e.g., "this headache will make it impossible for me to get anything done") and minimize the available psychosocial resources (e.g., "I cannot do anything to influence this headache," "no one can help me"). Other cognitive reactions fall into the errors-of-thinking categories outlined above that are associated with negative emotions, such as "these headaches will result in my losing my job" (catastrophizing).

Other cognitive reactions to headaches do not fit readily into the stress or negative emotions categories discussed so far but nevertheless appear maladaptive. For example, a common response to a headache is to question why it occurred. Of course, this reaction is consistent with the self-management approach advocated in this book: Patients should try to understand their headaches and learn lessons from headache attacks. On the other hand, headache sufferers often morbidly ruminate for extended periods of time on the cause of their headaches, and such a process is only likely to lead to an attentional focus on the pain and negative affect (e.g., tension, frustration, anger).

Many of the thoughts that occur following a headache are not in response to the headache per se but to associated factors. For example, consuming medication often leads to anxiety-provoking thoughts such as "will taking these drugs cause brain/kidney damage?" Accompanying symptoms such as nausea, photophobia, and vertigo can trigger negative thoughts.

Sometimes reactions to headaches can be divided into two or more distinct but interrelated phases. Common themes of a first phase are attempts to "fight" the headache or ignore it. If these coping efforts are unsuccessful, a second phase may be characterized by thoughts associated with anger, depression, or resignation.

Identifying and Challenging Maladaptive Thoughts

The procedures used for identifying and challenging both maladaptive thoughts and underlying assumptions are based on the work of Beck and his colleagues (e.g., Beck et al., 1979).

After discussing the rationale of the cognitive approach with patients, the next step is to help them identify maladaptive thoughts related to stress and headaches. This process begins with the therapist's using information from completed change cards to discuss maladaptive thoughts the patient has had in response to headaches. The process continues by patient self-monitoring using "maladaptive thoughts records."

MALADAPTIVE THOUGHTS RECORD

This form of diary is an adaptation of the Dysfunctional Thoughts Record (Beck et al., 1979). A completed example of the record is presented as Figure 11.1. The record pertains to one of the cases discussed in Chapter 8 (Clare).

The aim of the maladaptive thoughts record is to collect information about thoughts and feelings during the critical periods of high stress, negative emotions, headache onset, and severe headache. A balance needs to be found between asking patients to complete records often enough to capture significant details and overloading them with recording requirements. For this reason, the criteria used for completing maladaptive thoughts records must be individualized for each patient and may need adjustment if the criteria lead to too many or too few records. Some guidelines for setting criteria include the following:

1. *Elevated stress.* To avoid introducing patients to more new scales than is necessary, this criterion may be defined in terms of the 6-point stress scale that they have already used with the change and control cards. An exemplar criterion would be "complete a maladaptive thoughts record whenever you would rate your stress level as 3 or above." If patients tend to be unaware of their stress levels, one approach to this problem is to ask them to rate their level of stress hourly at the same time that they rate their headache intensity. These stress ratings can be recorded on the daily cards using a different symbol to the headache ratings (e.g., circles vs. crosses).

2. *Negative emotions.* A criterion for completing records on the basis of negative emotions can also be defined in terms of the previously used 6-point scale. On the other hand, the maladaptive thoughts record requires patients to rate emotions on a scale from 0 to 100 so that it is probably better to use a criterion such as "complete a record whenever you experience negative emotions at an intensity of 50 or higher."

3. *Headaches.* Patients should be asked to complete a maladaptive thoughts record whenever a headache begins or becomes severe. For defining severe, the daily cards should be consulted to determine what constitutes severe for that individual. A criterion that is often appropriate is to specify

DATE	STRESSOR	EMOTION(S)	SITUATION	MALADAPTIVE THOUGHTS	RATIONAL RESPONSES	OUTCOME
1. Day 2. Time	1. Stress (0-5) 2. Headache (0-5)	Feeling(s) and intensity (0-100)	Event, activity or general topic of thought	Actual thoughts and belief in each (0-100)	Responses to verbal challenging and belief in each (0-100)	1. Thoughts (0-100) 2. Emotion(s) (0-100) 3. Stress (0-5) 4. Headache (0-5)
1. 10/2/91 2. 6.30 pm	1. Stress (4) 2. Headache (3)	Anger (80) Tension (70)	Preparing dinner whilst feeding baby.	I am sick of having damn headaches. This headache will make the evening unbearable. If I ask my husband to help prepare the meal, he will refuse and be nasty to me (90).	My headaches are distressing but 'magnifying' the experience will only make them worse (90). If I can keep calm and reduce this headache, the evening may work out okay (75). My husband may be prepared to assist me, he sometimes has in the past (85). My husband may not be unpleasant to me (70). If my husband reacts by sighing or giving 'sideways' looks, it really isn't the end of the world (80).	1. Thoughts (60) 2. Anger (50) Tension (50) 3. Stress (2) 4. Headache (2)

FIGURE 11.1. Maladaptive thoughts record.

181

severe in terms of the two highest intensity ratings that the patient uses regularly.

The seven columns of the maladaptive thoughts record are completed as follows:

1. *Date*. Patients record the date and time of the recording.

2. *Stressor*. Patients rate their stress level and headache intensity using previously described six-point scales.

3. *Emotion(s)*. Patients are asked to list all the emotions that they are experiencing and to record after each one the intensity of the emotion on a scale from 0 to 100. A rating of 100 is defined as an emotion as strong as it could possibly be.

4. *Situation*. Patients are required to briefly describe the situation they were in (e.g., arguing with boss), or the general topic that they were thinking about (e.g., worrying about paying accounts due).

5. *Maladaptive thoughts*. Patients are asked to record their thoughts accurately, word for word. They are also requested to rate how far they believed each thought on a 0–100 scale, where 100 means that they are totally convinced.

6. *Rational responses*. Patients are trained to verbally challenge their maladaptive thoughts by asking a series of questions (see below). The responses to these questions are recorded in this column, together with ratings of the extent to which patients believe each response, as for maladaptive thoughts.

7. *Outcome*. The final column of the diary is used for recording the impact of the verbal challenging on the patient's belief in the maladaptive thoughts and his or her emotions, stress level, and headache intensity. The pre- and postchallenging ratings are carried out because it is unlikely that the challenging will lead to dramatic, immediate changes in thoughts, feelings, and sensations: The ratings enable small changes to be observed.

VERBAL CHALLENGING AND BEHAVIORAL EXPERIMENTS

The approach taken to challenging maladaptive thoughts is based on Fennell (1989). There are two main methods used for challenging maladaptive thoughts and generating more adaptive, coping patterns of thinking. Verbal challenging involves asking questions that address the validity of the maladaptive thoughts. Behavioral experiments involve testing new ideas in action.

Verbal challenging proceeds with the therapist encouraging the patient to evaluate his or her maladaptive thoughts via a series of questions, the first of which is, "What is the evidence?" In discussing this question with the patient, it is important for the therapist to be aware of the biases headache sufferers may display as a consequence of their pain or the negative emotions that frequently accompany headaches. Recent research findings suggest, for example, that anxiety is associated with attentional biases (anxious individuals selectively attend to threatening stimuli), anxiety and depression are associated with mood congruent interpretative biases, and depression is associated with recall biases (negatively valenced material is remembered relative to positively valenced material) (MacLeod & Mathews, 1991). Efforts should be made to uncover disconfirming evidence of which the patient is not initially aware and to challenge the validity of apparently negative evidence.

A second question for verbal challenging is, "What alternative views are there?" If patients experience difficulty answering the question in this form, variations can be used such as "What might someone else whose opinions you respect think about this?" or "What would you say to another person who expressed those thoughts?" A third useful question is, "What are the advantages and disadvantages of this way of thinking?" The final method of verbal challenging is to ask the question, "What logical errors am I making?" This question requires patients to analyze their maladaptive thoughts in terms of the seven errors in thinking discussed above.

Verbal challenging of maladaptive thoughts can be followed by behavioral experiments that test the validity of the answers to the questions (i.e., the rational responses). Fennell suggests five steps for setting up behavioral experiments:

1. *Prediction.* The first step involves specifying the maladaptive thoughts the experiment will test. Using the example in Figure 11.1, the thought to be tested might be, "If I ask my husband to help prepare the meal he will refuse and be nasty to me."

2. *Review.* The second step involves reviewing existing evidence for and against the prediction, and hence parallels the verbal challenging. Following through the above example, questions to be asked here include, "How has he behaved previously in this situation or similar situations (e.g., alternative problems to headache or alternative types of help requested)?"

3. *Design.* This step involves devising a specific experiment to test the validity of the prediction. Experiments should be set up so that it is clear exactly what the patient will do, and so as to maximize the chances of a positive outcome. In the example considered so far, how the patient asked her husband for help would be considered in detail, with role playing a possible option.

4. *Results.* The outcome of the experiment may be desirable (i.e., contrary to the maladaptive thought and consistent with the rational responses(s)) or undesirable (i.e., consistent with the maladaptive thought). If the former ocurs, the belief in the maladaptive thought should be weakened. If the latter occurs, the outcome of the experiment should be viewed as an

opportunity for learning by posing further questions, such as "What went wrong?" and "Was the experiment effectively sabotaged by further maladaptive thoughts?" Once the problem has been identified, plans can be made to cope with the situation more effectively in the future.

5. *Conclusions.* Finally, it can be helpful to formulate a rule summarizing what has been learned. For example, "Don't make assumptions about how other people will react, rather, take steps to find out."

Identifying and Challenging Maladaptive Beliefs

Once patients can identify and challenge maladaptive thoughts, the next phase of treatment involves focusing on the maladaptive beliefs or assumptions that underlie the thoughts. Beck, Hollon, Young, Bedrosian, and Budenz (1985) have categorized maladaptive assumptions in terms of three central areas of concern: (1) achievement (e.g., the need to succeed, perform well), (2) acceptance (e.g., the need to be liked, loved), and (3) control (e.g., the need to control events, be strong).

Maladaptive beliefs are more difficult to identify than maladaptive thoughts as they are generalized rules that may never have been formulated. They need to be inferred rather than observed, and Fennell lists six clues to aid in this process:

1. *Themes.* Themes may emerge during treatment that give clues to underlying assumptions. For example, a constant striving for success might suggest a belief such as, "I am inadequate unless I succeed."

2. *Logical errors.* Logical errors in maladaptive thoughts may reflect similar errors in maladaptive beliefs. For example, the maladaptive thought "I am a hopeless mother because my headaches have stopped my taking part in my children's school activities" (dichotomous reasoning) may be associated with the maladaptive belief that "health problems shouldn't interfere with any of one's roles or responsibilities."

3. *Global evaluations.* Global evaluations of self or others may give clues to underlying beliefs. For example, a self-description as "weak" may reflect a belief in the need to be strong.

4. *Early memories.* People sometimes have vivid memories of childhood experiences that seem to match current beliefs. For example, individuals with beliefs concerning the need to comply with all requests made of them may recall childhood experiences in which this belief was reinforced by statements to the effect that if they didn't do what they were told, some dire consequences would follow.

5. *Excessive emotions.* High mood often indicates that the terms of an assumption have been met; low mood signals the violation of the assumption. For example, a person who believes it is necessary always to be in control will

be devastated (rather than distressed) when a headache results in his or her having to cancel a commitment.

6. *Vertical arrow*. This technique was developed by Burns (1980) and initially involves identifying maladaptive thoughts in the usual way. Then, rather than challenging the thoughts, the therapist asks exploratory questions in the form, "Supposing that was true, what would that mean to you?" The technique involves asking such questions until it is possible to formulate a statement general enough to encompass not only the original problem situation but also other situations in which the same rule is operating. The name of the technique derives from the method of recording: A vertical arrow is drawn from the original maladaptive thought leading to the first question of the therapist; another vertical arrow leads from this question to the response, and so forth.

Once a maladaptive belief has been identified, it needs to be challenged via questioning and behavioral experiments. Fennell recommends four core questions for this purpose, the first two of which parallel verbal challenges to maladaptive thoughts. "In what way is the belief unreasonable?" calls for an assessment of the relevant evidence. The question involves considering whether the belief is consistent with the way the world works and the reality of human experience. For example, "I should always be strong" ignores human frailty.

A second useful question is, "In what way is the belief unhelpful?" A good method of approaching this question is to list the advantages and disadvantages of holding the belief. This often reveals that the latter outweigh the former. Perfectionist beliefs are often defended by patients, for example, on the ground that they lead to high-quality work. Listing disadvantages will emphasize associated drawbacks such as the excessive time devoted to achieving very small, additional gains and the anxiety such beliefs engender, leading to avoidance of opportunities.

A third question is, "Where did the belief come from?" Understanding how maladaptive beliefs were formed can help patients distance themselves from the beliefs. They often can appreciate that beliefs formed in early life are no longer applicable to their current circumstances.

A final useful question is, "What would be a more moderate alternative belief that would confer the advantages of the maladaptive belief without its disadvantages?" Maladaptive beliefs are usually rigid, overgeneralized, and extreme in their demands. Formulating an alternative that takes into account shades of gray prepares the person to deal effectively with occasions that, in terms of the original belief, would count as failures and lead to negative affect. Alternatives to maladaptive beliefs can be written on "flash cards" that consist of a statement of the belief followed by rational responses to the belief and a plan for change (Clark & Beck, 1988). Patients are required to read the flash card repeatedly until acting in accordance with it becomes automatic.

Verbal challenging to maladaptive beliefs can be followed up by behavioral experiments. Given the likelihood that beliefs are long standing, behavioral experiments that target beliefs may need to be repeated over a more extended period and in a wider variety of situations than behavioral experiments that target thoughts. Behavioral experiments can take a number of forms, including (1) gathering information about other people's standards rather than assuming one's own are universal, (2) observing what others do as an indication of their differing standards, (3) acting contrary to assumptions and observing the consequences, and (4) testing the new rule in action.

Focus on Antecedents

Immediate Factors

The assessment of immediate antecedents by interview, questionnaires, self-monitoring, and behavioral experiments was discussed in Chapter 7. Evidence was reviewed in Chapter 4 suggesting that simply encouraging migraineurs to avoid precipitating factors can reduce headaches (Blau & Thavapalan, 1988; Dalton, 1973). The most common immediate antecedents of headaches are stress and negative emotions. The treatment approach discussed in the previous section addresses these factors.

FOOD AND FASTING

Some authors have advocated particular types of diets for headache sufferers, such as a tyramine-free diet (Diamond, 1979) or a monosodium glutamate-free diet (Scopp, 1991). These approaches seem less than ideal, however, because so many different foods are potentially capable of inducing headaches (see Chapter 4) and headaches are triggered by different foods for different individuals. Also, the only controlled trial of a standard diet approach to headaches failed to show its efficacy (Medina & Diamond, 1978).

The approach that seems more sound logically and better supported empirically is the use of an individualized elimination diet regime (Grant, 1979; O'Banion, 1981). Different authors have proposed variations on this method which, in essence, involve first placing patients on a restricted diet that is unlikely to precipitate headaches, and second, reintroducing foods one at a time while testing the effects. For the restricted diet, Grant has recommended that patients eat only two low-risk foods (usually lamb and pears) and drink bottled spring water for 5 days; O'Banion suggests that patients eat only fresh meats, vegetables, and fruit and drink tap water. Raskin (1988) advocates distilled water (for cooking, drinking, and brushing the teeth), lamb, rice, and boiled or baked potatoes, for a period dependent on the frequency of headache attacks.

If the restricted diet leads to a reduction in headaches, a testing phase is implemented during which foods are reintroduced one at a time and their effects monitored by recording headache activity following consumption. If consumption of specific foods is associated with headache symptoms, the food is either eliminated from the diet or subsequently retested.

Another dietary principle for headaches is the need for a "diversified rotating" diet (Grant, 1979; O'Banion, 1981). It is argued that this prevents food allergies from developing.

In addition to food causing headaches, it is noted in Chapter 4 that fasting seems to be a common precipitator of headaches. The length of time an individual can manage without food while leading an active life varies considerably (Dalton, 1973). Men can last longer than women, and women are particularly vulnerable during their paramenstrum. Patients who suffer from headaches triggered by fasting obviously should be counseled about the need to avoid missing meals or delayed meals. Dalton advocates snacks between meals for such individuals or dividing three meals into six snacks. In a similar vein, Raskin (1988) recommends trying a high-protein, low-carbohydrate multiple feeding schedule. "Sunday-morning headaches" may arise from eating breakfast late, and this can be avoided either by having a snack just before going to bed the night before or by having a snack available by the bedside to eat or drink at the regular breakfast time.

PERCEPTUAL STIMULI

Many patients report that a range of visual stimuli including flicker, glare, and eyestrain will precipitate or aggravate their headaches. Conditions such as bright sunlight, fluorescent light, and observing television or computer screens can trigger headaches. Patients often become more sensitive to visual discomfort during headaches.

Most of the visual conditions associated with headaches are amenable to change. Patients who are vulnerable to headaches caused by bright sunlight and glare can be encouraged to avoid going outside when extreme conditions prevail, or to wear a hat and sunglasses. Internal lighting conditions can sometimes be modified by replacing fluorescent lights with incandescent lights and decreasing or increasing levels of illumination depending on whether the problem is too much or too little light. If internal lighting cannot be changed, patients can be encouraged to wear tinted or polarized lenses to counteract fluorescent light and glare. Rose-colored tinted glasses have been shown to reduce the frequency of migraine attacks in children (Good, Taylor, & Mortimer, 1991). Eyestrain can be reduced by avoiding activities that lead to it or scheduling activities differently (e.g., multiple short exposures rather than single long exposures).

On the other hand, a laboratory study by Philips and Jahanshahi (1985) raises the issue of whether avoidance of perceptual stimuli that induce headaches may make headache sufferers less tolerant of the stimuli. These authors evaluated the efficacy of four exposure conditions on tolerance for noise stimuli: (1) short exposure, (2) long exposure, (3) long exposure under conditions of relaxation, and (4) no exposure. They found that avoidance of noise stimuli was associated with decreased tolerance for the stimuli while exposure to noise stimuli was associated with increased tolerance. Long exposure under conditions of relaxation was most effective in increasing tolerance.

This study suggests that an appropriate treatment for headaches induced by noise stimuli would be long exposure to noise stimuli under relaxation conditions, as this would desensitize patients to the nociceptive qualities of the stimuli. The same argument could be applied to visual stimuli. Such strategies have not been reported in the literature, however, so it is still an open question whether the pragmatic approach of avoidance with the attendant risk of increasing sensitivity or an exposure-based approach is more advantageous.

OTHER FACTORS

Many other situations and conditions that precipitate or aggravate headaches are amenable to modification. A good example is the fatigue arising from exertion or lack of sleep which often triggers headaches. Addressing the issues that have led to these conditions can reduce their occurrence. Teaching patients to reorganize their schedules and commitments, for example, can pay dividends in this respect. For headaches that are precipitated or aggravated by smoking, efforts aimed at helping sufferers to reduce or abandon smoking are appropriate (Payne et al., 1991).

Many medications are capable of exacerbating headaches, including nitroglycerin, hydralazine, reserpine, vitamin A, clomiphene, and indomethacin (Raskin, 1988). Requesting physicians to review such medications and eliminate or change the drugs if there is any suspicion that they are aggravating the headache problem is recommended.

Setting Factors

STRESS

One approach to stress-related headaches is to focus on the major sources of stress. A common cause of distress is family relationships, and a variety of forms of intervention may be appropriate. For difficulties arising from parenting, training in child management skills (Dangel & Polster, 1988) may be helpful. Marital therapy (Jacobson & Gurman, 1986) or family therapy (Falloon, 1988) might be the most appropriate approach if the difficulties lie in the relationship with the partner or are more broadly based within the family system. Problems may exist in the extended family with parents, in-laws, brothers and sisters, and so forth. If relatives are unable or unwilling to attend therapy, teaching the patient personal skills related to relationships, such as social skills (L'Abate & Milan, 1985) and assertion skills (Lange & Jakubowski, 1976), may be the most helpful form of intervention.

Stress evolving from sources such as career, finances, and housing can be addressed via counseling whether this is carried out by the therapist or through referral to another service provider. A common stressor in headache sufferers is ruminations about unfulfilling life situations and lack of plans for the future. Such problems can be addressed by counseling to help patients understand their full range of options and make decisions about directions they wish to follow.

An alternative approach to stress-related headaches is to focus on the variables that mediate the stress response. A previous section discussed cognitive techniques that target appraisal and coping processes. Because social support can act as a buffer against stress (Peterson, 1991), training aimed at teaching headache sufferers to mobilize social support can be beneficial (Parry, 1988). In a review of support interventions, Gottlieb (1988) argues that deficiencies in individual social skills may detract from the support individuals receive, but also recent research has shown that certain ways of coping invite support while other ways inhibit support. Dunkel-Schetter, Folkman, and Lazarus (1987), for example, found that problem-solving modes of coping (making a plan of action and solving it) elicited more support of all types than did palliative modes (distancing oneself from the problem or from feelings about it). Gottlieb also emphasizes that individuals are more likely to receive support if they control their own experience of distress during supportive exchanges.

NEGATIVE EMOTIONS

If headaches are strongly related to negative emotions such as anxiety, depression, and anger, then treatments targeting emotional states may be warranted. Some of the techniques already discussed are used in the treatment of negative affect. Relaxation training and cognitive approaches focusing on changing maladaptive thoughts and beliefs are treatment methods employed for anxiety, for example. Other anxiety management methods may also be useful. Techniques in which patients are exposed to anxiety-inducing stimuli are widely used in the treatment of anxiety disorders (Barlow, 1988) and can be relevant for headache sufferers. Headaches triggered by anxiety-provoking situations such as social situations and agoraphobic-type situations, for example, can be treated via exposure methods. Payne and Colletti (1991) provide an illustration of the successful application of this approach in their report of an adolescent girl whose headaches failed to respond to progressive relaxation and assertion training, but who achieved a substantial reduction in headaches via implosive therapy focusing on an episode of sexual abuse.

The previously discussed cognitive approaches targeting maladaptive thoughts and beliefs are also relevant to depression, but other techniques developed for treating depression can be useful for headaches associated with depressed mood. Behavioral strategies such as mastery and pleasure technique, scheduling activities, and graded task assignment are all potentially useful approaches, particularly for withdrawn headache sufferers who are inactive (Beck et al., 1979).

The most established approach to the regulation of anger has been developed by Novaco (e.g., Novaco, 1979). Nocavo uses a stress inoculation model with three phases: cognitive preparation, skill acquisition, and application training. This approach overlaps methods already discussed (e.g., it includes cognitive techniques similar to those previously considered, and includes relaxation training) and is a variation of a model that has also been applied to other clinical problems including anxiety (Meichenbaum, 1975) and pain (Turk, 1976).

LIFE-STYLE APPROACHES

A number of aspects of life-style seem relevant to headache management. Saper (1989) has argued that "migraine prone patients seem to fare better with regularity established in primary life functions" (p. 391). Hence, he advocates promoting "sameness" from day to day in terms of sleeping patterns, eating habits, and so forth. Exercise is associated with many health benefits, including a number of psychological effects that may be advantageous to headache sufferers such as decreased depression, tension, and anxiety and improved self-concept (Dubbert, Martin, & Epstein, 1986). Several studies have reported on the benefits of exercise as a treatment for headaches (e.g., Grimm, Douglas, & Hanson, 1981; Hage, 1981; Lockett & Campbell, 1992). Spending time engaged in leisure activities can serve as a distraction from routine concerns or anxiety-provoking situations and provide mastery and pleasure experiences that protect against depression. Exercise and leisure activities that involve social interaction can also lead to increased social networks with associated stress-buffering benefits. Training in the principles of time management can be beneficial (Clark, 1989) to headache sufferers who lead a life-style characterized by intense time pressure. Training in problem solving

(Hawton & Kirk, 1989) can help headache sufferers manage a range of personal issues.

RELATED PROBLEMS

Headache sufferers sometimes present with problems in addition to their headaches, such as low back pain, insomnia, and overweight, which interact with their headache disorder. For example, low back pain constitutes a stressor and can lead to negative affect such as anxiety and depression and family conflict, thus creating conditions conducive to headaches. Insomnia often provides headache sufferers with the opportunity to ruminate about their headaches and can result in chronic tiredness and low mood. Obesity can lead to reduced activity, depression, and lowered self-esteem.

If conditions such as these seem to play an important role in the headache problem, it is worth considering whether the conditions should be treated prior to, or concurrently with, treatment of the headache problem.

Onset and Predisposing Factors

As noted in Chapter 9, consideration of onset factors is not likely to generate treatment strategies. If onset of headaches was associated with using oral contraceptives and the patient continued to use oral contraceptives, discontinuation for a period, and noting the effect on headaches, should be considered. In the case of headache onset associated with stressful and traumatic events, consideration of the original circumstances under which the headache developed may affect the stress management features of the treatment program (e.g., gives clues as to maladaptive beliefs).

With respect to predisposing factors, a number of personality characteristics or behavioral styles that seem to make patients vulnerable to developing headaches or other stress-related problems may be suitable targets for treatment. Some personality features appear likely to predispose individuals to find a variety of situations stressful. Perfectionism, for example, results in high standards that are likely to be violated. Rigidity acts as a constraint on the ability to cope effectively with different demands. A high need for being in control creates problems given the difficulty or impossibility of controlling some situations. Personality characteristics such as these are likely to be addressed via the cognitive approach focusing on maladaptive thoughts and beliefs, given that these characteristics will manifest in broad beliefs.

Individuals who are high on trait anxiety, anger, or depression would seem at increased risk of headaches triggered by these emotions. Treatment aimed at anxiety, anger, and depression has been discussed in previous sections.

A number of other personality features that make individuals vulnerable to stress-related headaches could be treated by techniques discussed already. For example, patients low on assertiveness, or unable to express their emotions, should benefit from assertion training. Patients with poor communication skills would benefit from marital therapy if the communication problem involved the partner, given that marital therapy includes communication training.

A behavioral style that might be an appropriate target for intervention with headache sufferers is the Type A personality. Roskies (1983) has developed a stress management program for Type A individuals with the following components: (1) progressive relaxation, (2) rational–emotive therapy adapted for focus on anger, (3) communication skills training, (4) problem solving, and (5) stress inoculation training adapted for focus on time pressure. Again, this program overlaps treatments already considered but includes some different elements.

Personality characteristics that can set people up for stress-related headaches and other problems include low self-esteem and low self-confidence. Programs have been developed for enhancing self-esteem that use cognitive techniques to change self-critical thoughts and underlying beliefs and imagery techniques to improve self-image (McKay & Fanning, 1987).

Focus on Consequences

Immediate Reactions

REACTIONS OF SUFFERERS

Techniques targeting maladaptive cognitive reactions to headaches were discussed earlier in this chapter. Such an approach is based on the assumption that changing thoughts will result in changes in associated feelings (e.g., anxiety, anger, frustration) and behavior (e.g., belligerent and aggressive acts) which will break down stress–headache–stress vicious cycles. In addition to these reactions to headaches as stressors, patients may respond in other ways that exacerbate antecedents or pain perception. For example, some headache sufferers respond to the possibility of a headache's developing or to headache onset by markedly increased activity so as to complete tasks before they are incapacitated by the headache. Such reactions created demands that seem likely to increase the probability of a headache's developing or becoming more severe. These responses can be modified by a combination of cognitive and behavioral strategies. Patients should be encouraged to consider alternative reactions to their headaches and to consider the advantages and disadvantages associated with each. Behavioral assignments can be set whereby patients are asked to explore alternative forms of response.

Some behavioral reactions to headaches are extreme in the opposite direction to the one just described: Patients take medication and sit or lie down. This reaction could lead to the adverse consequences associated with avoidance behavior described by Philips (1987a) as a reduction in the sufferer's belief in his or her ability to control pain and described by Lethem et al. (1983) as reinforcement of "invalid status." On the other hand, whether this reaction can be classified as maladaptive is debatable. Anyone who has experienced a severe migraine attack would not argue with the proposition that resorting to medication and rest is sometimes necessary. The danger with chronic headache sufferers is in developing a tendency to overreact, and to respond in this way when it is not necessary. As with the increased activity response to headaches, this reaction should be discussed with the patient in the context of alternatives. The patient should be encouraged to experiment in order to gain further information and to discover the most appropriate response for him or her.

An issue that arises with many headache sufferers is whether they should inform others when they have a headache. Many adopt extreme reactions, either never telling anyone or always telling everyone within hearing. The former has the disadvantage that if others do not know when the sufferer is experiencing a headache, they cannot offer support or help in any way; the latter has the disadvantage that others are likely to react negatively if they view the sufferer as someone who is constantly complaining. Again, patients need to be encouraged to consider the advantages and disadvantages of their way of reacting to headaches and alternatives and to explore different ways of responding.

A common response of sufferers to their headaches is to take medication. Medication consumption may be excessive in the sense of being potentially damaging physiologically or being liable to induce headaches. Alternatively, consumption may simply exceed the patient's desired levels. Reduction of prescribed medication should obviously be accomplished with medical collaboration. Decreases in nonprescription drugs can be achieved by a gradual reduction process as treatment progresses. Baumgartner et al. (1989) have pointed out, however, that drug-induced headaches are difficult to treat for several reasons, including (1) physical and psychological dependence, (2) ineffectiveness of standard prophylactic medications with these cases, and (3) withdrawal headaches, often accompanied by a number of unpleasant symptoms (e.g., nausea, vomiting, mood, and sleep disturbances), caused by discontinuance of analgesics.

REACTIONS OF OTHERS

If reinforcement mechanisms appear to be maintaining headaches, contingency management procedures are called for. It was noted in Chapter 7 that it
is difficult to determine whether reinforcement mechanisms are operative.
Carrying out contingency management programs with headache sufferers is
also problematic. The published literature provides limited guidelines because application to headaches is largely restricted to two case studies describing these methods used with children (reviewed in Chapter 4) and a few
suggestive paragraphs (e.g, Adams, 1985). Fordyce provides a quite detailed
description of this approach in his book (Fordyce, 1976), but his methods
were developed with chronic low back pain patients. The characteristics of
headache sufferers are quite different from those of low back pain sufferers
and necessitate revision of his procedures for application to headache patients.

Contingency management methods require control of the patient's environment. Fordyce achieves an approximation to this control by admitting
chronic pain patients to a special ward for an average period of 8 weeks (range
4–19 weeks) followed by 4 weeks of outpatient treatment (Fowler, 1975). It is
difficult to justify extended hospitalizations such as these for headache sufferers given that most are not disabled by their headaches. Consequently,
contingency management procedures must be implemented by training relatives to carry out the program. This is not simple.

The core principles of Fordyce's approach are to minimize the reinforcement of pain behavior while maximizing the reinforcement of well behavior.
Consideration of the application of these principles to headache sufferers
raises a number of issues. For example, extinction of all pain behavior such as
verbal reports of headaches seems an inappropriate treatment goal as requesting help can be adaptive. To suggest to an individual that if his or her partner
were experiencing a severe migraine attack accompanied by vertigo, nausea,
and vomiting the individual should be "socially unresponsive," to avoid
reinforcing headaches, seems equally inappropriate. On the other hand, if
even mild headaches are consistently followed by positive reinforcement
(e.g., attention, sympathy, interest) and negative reinforcement (e.g., avoidance of unappealing tasks and events), modification of consequences seems
appropriate. Hence, negotiation has to take place between the therapist,
patient, and relatives with respect to appropriate reactions by the relatives to
knowledge that the patient is experiencing a headache.

The principle of rewarding well behavior is implemented with back pain
sufferers by simply shaping up activity levels. This seems inappropriate with
most headache sufferers as most are quite active between headaches and even
during minor headaches. On the other hand, the principle has application in
a revised form. Headache sufferers sometimes avoid certain activities and
events in case participation might lead to headaches, even when the evidence

that this will happen is limited or nonexistent. In such instances, relatives can be encouraged to reinforce headache patients for nonavoidance.

Perhaps the most appropriate way of conceptualizing contingency management procedures applied to headache sufferers is for relatives to be trained to shape appropriate coping behaviors. As noted previously, lying on a bed may be the most appropriate response to a severe headache, and avoiding certain high-risk events or situations may also be appropriate. Other complaint or avoidance responses that seem maladaptive should not be followed by reinforcement, while use of coping strategies such as relaxation and imagery techniques should be reinforced.

Training of relatives starts with an explanation of the potential role of reinforcement in chronic headache problems. This is a difficult topic to discuss with patients and their families as there is a tendency for the explanation to be interpreted as implying that the headaches are not genuine in some way but simply a strategy to gain rewards. Care must be taken to emphasize that this is not the case and that learning can take place without awareness.

Training proceeds by defining key behavioral terms and principles such as positive reinforcement, negative reinforcement, social unresponsiveness (which is differentiated from ignoring), punishment, schedules of reinforcement, shaping, extinction, and generalization. Negotiations need to take place with respect to how the relatives should respond to different behaviors of the patient. Role playing is a useful technique for teaching appropriate responses.

Again, it is not an easy task to get relatives to change their behavior in accordance with the objectives of the program. Their responses have usually been established over long periods. Also, many spouses find it difficult to be socially unresponsive when their partners are experiencing some pain.

One very important point to establish in contingency management programs is that the overall level of reinforcement should not decline. While reinforcement is being withdrawn for certain types of pain behavior, it should be increased for more adaptive, coping behavior, resulting in the overall balance remaining the same or increasing. Sometimes headache sufferers only get support and assistance from their partners when they have a headache, so there is a danger that reducing reinforcement for pain behavior will leave them with no support at all.

Long-Term Effects

Little needs to be said about the treatment of the long-term effects of headaches, as the effects that may arise overlap focuses for treatment described in previous sections. For example, chronic headaches lead to decreased feelings of self-efficacy with respect to headaches and a reduced sense of control over pain. Targeting these cognitive changes was discussed in the first section of this chapter. Headaches can lead to both intrapersonal and interpersonal problems such as depression, insomnia, and marital distress. Headaches can also give rise to reduced leisure activities and exercise and decreased social support. All these problems can constitute setting factors for headaches, and hence treatment focusing on them has already been discussed. Headaches can detrimentally affect personality features such as self-esteem and self-confidence. Treatment targeting these characteristics was considered in the predisposing factors section.

Treatment Summary

Treatment techniques that are appropriate for use with most chronic headache cases are listed in Table 11.1. An educational component is the

TABLE 11.1. Treatment Techniques Appropriate for Most Chronic Headache Cases

Treatment techniques	Commencing session

Education
  Intervention model
  Functional model of chronic headaches
  Model of patient's headaches
  Treatment program
	Session 3 or 4

Relaxation training
  Progressive relaxation (recommended)
  Autogenic training (alternative)
  Behavioral relaxation training (alternative)
	Session 4 or 5

Cognitive training
  Identifying and challenging
  • Maladaptive thoughts
  • Maladaptive beliefs
	Session 5 or 6

Imagery training
  Incompatible imagery
  • Emotive imagery
  • Sensory imagery
  Transformative imagery
  • Contextual imagery
  • Stimulus imagery
  • Response imagery
	Clinical judgment

Attention–diversion training
  Internal attention–diversion
  • Mental activity
  • Bodily process and sensations
  External attention–diversion
  • Features of environment
  • Distracting activities
	Clinical judgment

obvious starting point for a treatment program. For most patients I recommend that relaxation training commence in the following session. This approach has good face validity for the treatment of headaches and is easy for patients to follow. I have suggested progressive relaxation as the relaxation technique of choice, but for a number of reasons the therapist might start with a different method, or change to a different method, including the following: (1) the patient has tried progressive relaxation previously and had a negative experience (e.g., caused pain or was not successful), (2) there are problems

TABLE 11.2. Treatment Techniques Appropriate for Chronic Headaches with Particular Controlling Variables

Immediate antecedents	
Food	Elimination diet
Fasting	Frequent (high-protein, low-carbohydrate) food intake
Perceptual stimuli	Strategies designed to reduce or eliminate extreme visual and noise stimuli (or exposure-based treatment)
Other factors	Strategies aimed at reducing fatigue or eliminating headache-inducing medication, etc.
Setting antecedents	
Stress	Treatment focused on sources of stress (e.g., child management training, marital therapy, family therapy, assertion training, social skills training, vocational counseling) or aimed at increasing perceived social support
Negative emotions	Treament focused on anxiety, depression, and anger
Life-style approaches	Techniques aimed at establishing regular routines, engaging in leisure activities and regular exercise
Related problems	Treatment targeting associated problems such as low back pain, insomnia, and overweight
Onset and predisposing antecedents	
Personality characteristics	Interventions aimed at modifying personality features that make headache sufferers vulnerable to stress-related headaches: • Personality factors that set up an individual for experiencing situations as stressful (e.g., perfectionism, rigidity, need for control) • High trait anxiety, anger, and depression • Type A personality • Low self-esteem and low self-confidence
Immediate reactions	
Reactions of sufferers	Modification of maladaptive behavioral reactions (e.g., overactive or underactive, taking excessive medication)
Reactions of others	Contingency management procedures directed toward relatives shaping up appropriate coping behaviors
Long-term effects	
Long-term consequences	Techniques aimed at reversing the effects of chronic headaches, such as decreased self-efficacy; depression, insomnia, and marital distress; reduced leisure activities, exercise, and perceived social support; and lowered self-esteem

associated with performing the tension-release cycles (e.g., difficulty releasing tension), and (3) the patient does not like or respond to progressive relaxation.

Cognitive training focusing on maladaptive thoughts and underlying beliefs should begin in the following session. It is probably worthwhile to train patients in some additional cognitive techniques (i.e., imagery and attention–diversion strategies), although whether it is appropriate to cover all nine variations depends on the particular case. Based on the research literature and clinical experience, I suggest the following cognitive strategies as the most suitable for use with chronic headache sufferers: incompatible sensory imagery (or imaginative inattention), stimulus transformation imagery, and response transformation imagery (or relabeling).

Treatment techniques predicated by the controlling variables of headaches are listed in Table 11.2. It is a matter of clinical judgment deciding which techniques to use and when to introduce them. There are a few obvious guidelines to follow in making such decisions: (1) how strong is the evidence that the hypothesized controlling variable is a factor in the headache problem (e.g., research findings relevant to the controlling variable, quality and consistency of assessment data), (2) how important a factor is the controlling variable (i.e., what percentage of the variance does it account for), (3) what is the likelihood that the controlling variable can be changed, and (4) what is the likely outcome of modifying the controlling variable on the headaches and other factors, both pertaining to the sufferer and significant others.

12

Case Examples of Psychological Treatment from a Functional Perspective

Case I: Clare

The patient, Clare, whose case was discussed in Chapter 8 and whose headaches were presented diagrammatically in Figure 8.1, was seen for a total of 15 sessions. The first 10 sessions were scheduled weekly except for a 2-week gap between weeks 5 and 6 due to illness, and the latter 5 sessions were scheduled every 2 weeks. Treatment sessions followed the format described in Chapter 9 of review, treatment techniques, and setting homework assignments. Summarized below are the treatment plan, process of treatment, and treatment outcome.

Treatment Plan

The following techniques constituted the treatment plan:

1. Education
2. Relaxation training (progressive relaxation)
3. Cognitive training focusing on maladaptive thoughts and beliefs
4. Imagery training
5. Attention–diversion training
6. Modification of immediate antecedents
7. Child management training
8. Modification of life-style aimed at increasing hobbies and interests
9. Modification of maladaptive behavioral reactions to headaches

10. Contingency management procedures targeting husband's responses to headaches

Process of Treatment

PRIOR TO FIRST APPOINTMENT, AND SESSIONS 1 AND 2

Clare was given the Preassessment Patient Information Sheet (Appendix 1) to read in the waiting room before the first appointment. An assessment interview was carried out across Sessions 1 and 2 following the format of the PAHQ as described in Chapter 6. At the end of Session 1 Clare was taught how to complete the daily cards. She was asked to start completing the cards on the first hour following the session and to continue with these records until 2 weeks after treatment ended. Clare was given a BDI and STAI and was requested to complete them the following morning and return the inventories at the next session. The results of these assessments are discussed in Chapter 8.

SESSION 3

This session was devoted to the educational component. Clare's husband, Jim, was invited to attend the session in view of his role in the proposed contingency management procedures. The session followed the four-stage sequence outlined in Chapter 9. The model of Clare's headaches presented in this session was similar to the one in Figure 8.1, although the one in Figure 8.1 includes revisions that mainly evolved from this session (i.e., feedback from Clare and Jim) and subsequent completion of change and control cards. Jim suggested that their children were active but within the normal range of variation and that the problems between them and Clare resulted from her unrealistic expectations and sensitivities. Although Clare was an intelligent and educated person, she showed little insight into her headaches and was reluctant to accept a role for reinforcement processes.

The session concluded with Clare's being taught how to complete the change and control cards. Clare and Jim were told that the first stage of the treatment program (three sessions) would involve teaching Clare some basic skills related to managing stress and headaches. Then Jim would be asked to attend again for setting up contingency management procedures.

SESSION 4

The review at the beginning of this session revealed that Jim had had flu during the week. Clare thought he "overreacted" to his symptoms "as he always did." This event had resulted in Clare's and Jim's reversing roles in terms of who was the sufferer, so some time was spent discussing what had occurred in order to increase Clare's understanding of how others might think and feel about her headaches. For example, Clare was asked about how she came to the conclusion that Jim overreacted. Also, she was asked to consider why Jim responded to her headaches as he did, taking into account her reaction to his illness behavior.

The main part of this session was devoted to relaxation training. Clare's only previous experience in relaxation training was a few group antenatal classes using a technique that sounded similar to progressive relaxation, and it had been a positive experience. Progressive relaxation training proceeded by outlining the rationale and then going through the tension-release cycles with the 16 muscle groups (Table 10.1). The training went well and Clare indicated that she was succeeding in releasing the various muscle groups, which was consistent with observation of her progress.

The session concluded with instructions to practice relaxation at home twice daily and to record details of the practice, as outlined in Chapter 10. Clare was provided with an audiotape of relaxation instructions and asked to use it for all practices for the first few days and then to use it for every other practice. Clare was also asked to complete the change and control cards for one more week.

SESSION 5

Inspection of home practice records at the beginning of the session indicated that when Clare practiced relaxation, it was leading to increased relaxation although the change was not as marked as had occurred in the office session. Clare was not practicing every day, however. When asked about this, she claimed that she was too busy on some days. It was pointed out to her with the aid of the daily cards that these tended to be the days on which she experienced more headache activity, and as such were particularly important days to practice.

The session proceeded by going through the tension-release cycles with seven muscle groups. The remainder of the session was spent on cognitive training for identifying and challenging maladaptive thoughts and beliefs. The rationale was covered and material from the last 2 weeks of completed change and control cards was used to provide examples of her maladaptive thinking. The homework assignment set was to complete the maladaptive thoughts records (note Figure 11.1 is an example of one record completed by Clare). Clare was requested to discontinue the change and control cards but to continue the relaxation practice using the seven muscle groups and a revised audiotape.

SESSION 6

Review of the homework assignments revealed that Clare had done a good job of identifying maladaptive thoughts but had not grasped the technique of verbal challenging. When she detected maladaptive thoughts she tended to distract herself rather than challenge them. The first part of the session was used for reviewing verbal challenging and behavioral experiments.

The second part of the session focused on immediate antecedents of headaches other than stress and negative affect. Food was largely ignored as the evidence for food's playing a significant role was generally not strong because Clare would make an observation on one occasion and then avoid the food. An exception was nuts, which were associated with headaches on a number of occasions, so Clare was encouraged not to eat nuts. Fasting had consistently led to headaches. Clare was encouraged to regularly consume high-protein, low-carbohydrate foods (i.e., meat, fish, eggs). Of course, since she was aware of an association between fasting and headaches she already tried to avoid delayed and missed meals, but she did not follow these strategies consistently. Clare was seen during summer/autumn, so the precipitating factor of cold winds never occurred. As heat and strong sunlight triggered headaches, she was encouraged to avoid these conditions or to take appropriate steps to minimize them.

The final part of the session focused on maladaptive behavioral reactions to headaches. Clare was discouraged from spring cleaning in response to headaches and encouraged to engage in strategies that would limit headaches as much as possible (e.g., relaxation, having a hot shower, or lying down). Clare believed that the children were a key problem in this respect because they hassled her and made it difficult for her to adopt some coping strategies. Discussion took place with respect to how she could get the children off her hands if she really needed to do so. She had local family who could look after the children, but she felt guilty asking them. Further discussion resulted in the conclusion that if she offered to help the relatives more, she would feel less guilty about asking them to care for the children.

For homework, Clare was asked to focus on minimizing headache triggers and to respond to headaches in more adaptive ways. She was requested to continue with the maladaptive thoughts records but to have a break from the relaxation practice.

SESSION 7

Jim had been invited to this session because its aim was to set up contingency management procedures. The session began with a discussion of the role of learning processes in chronic pain problems and key behavioral concepts, as outlined in Chapter 11. Discussion then turned to the specific aspects of Clare's case. It was noted that some of Jim's reactions to Clare's headaches could constitute positive reinforcement (e.g., coming home from work) and negative reinforcement (e.g., taking over the children). It was emphasized that it was appropriate to react in these ways if Clare really needed the support. On the other hand, the maximum intensity rating that Clare had used on the daily cards was 3 ("a painful headache, but one during which you could continue at your job") and the only accompanying symptom that sometimes occurred was nausea. In other words, Clare's headaches were an aversive experience but not exactly catastrophic events; the problem was more one of frequency (up to four a day) than of intensity. Discussion focused on the need for Jim to be more supportive, with his assistance not being dependent on Clare's complaining about headaches.

Jim was also asked to reinforce well behavior. Specifically, he should reinforce Clare when she agreed to take part in activities she had been avoiding on the grounds that they might precipitate headaches. He should also reinforce Clare when she used adaptive coping methods for managing stress and headaches, such as the skills she was learning through the treatment program (i.e., relaxation and cognitive strategies).

Discussion also took place with respect to what Clare didn't like about Jim's reactions to her headaches (e.g., his accusatory attitude, the way he took over the children but was lousy about it). To balance the discussion, Jim was also encouraged to talk about Clare's reactions to him when he suffered from problems, using the flu episode discussed in Session 4 as an example. The aim of this discussion was to give Clare and Jim more insight into each other's perspectives and to encourage them to adopt less punitive ways of responding to distress signals.

For homework, Clare was asked to continue with the maladaptive thoughts records and resume relaxation practice. Jim was asked to modify his behavior in accordance with the agreements reached in the session. He was told that he would be requested to attend another session in a few weeks time to review progress but meanwhile he was welcome to phone me or arrange to come to see me if he had any questions or ran into any problems.

SESSION 8

Review of the previous week suggested that the contingency management approach was going well. Clare indicated that Jim's attitude to her headaches had improved following Session 3 (education) and this improvement increased after the last session. She hadn't called him at work and only asked for help once in response to headaches. He had volunteered assistance on a number of occasions and reinforced her for using coping skills.

Relaxation training continued with tension-release cycles using four muscle groups. The remainder of the session was spent focusing on the maladaptive thoughts records. Clare had progressed from reacting to maladaptive thoughts by distracting herself to challenging the thoughts and devising appropriate behavioral experiments. For example, the spring cleaning response to headaches was driven by thoughts such as, "This house is such a mess and it will get worse while I have a headache." She was able to counter this type of thought via verbal challenging (e.g., "What is the evidence—has anyone ever suggested that my house looks a mess?") and behavioral experiments (e.g., asking other people whether they think her house ever looks a mess, and observing other people's houses). Beliefs underlying the maladaptive thoughts began to emerge, such as in the above example, "If my house isn't always perfectly tidy, then I am a failure as a housewife and therefore as a person."

Homework consisted of continuing with the maladaptive thoughts records and practicing relaxation with four muscle groups using a revised audiotape.

SESSION 9

The aim of this session was to cover techniques related to setting factors, namely, child management training and increasing hobbies and interests. With respect to the former, training started with a discussion of the degree to which the problem reflected her thoughts, beliefs, and feelings (e.g., unrealistic expectations, overly harsh judgments, anger driving her behavior) versus the behavior of the children. Clare was reminded that Jim had favored the former explanation in Session 3. Evidence supporting the role of such factors had arisen in the maladaptive thoughts records. One record completed when Clare felt stressed, for example, included maladaptive thoughts such as "Simon always wants to be the center of attention." On reviewing the evidence related to this thought, she realized that the statement was an exaggeration. Inspection of the maladaptive thoughts records suggested underlying beliefs such as, "Children should always be well behaved."

In addition to this cognitive approach to child management training, Clare's attention was drawn to the behavioral principles discussed in Session 7 as providing guidelines for regulating the behavior of her children. These principles were explained again in terms of their application to children rather than to adults. For example, time-out was discussed as a procedure for stopping serious misbehavior.

The nature of the problems with the children was discussed and how the behavioral principles could be applied to them. For example, Clare claimed that the children were overly demanding of her attention. Discussion of this issue revealed that Clare had labeled them as overly demanding and in reaction to this perception had increasingly avoided giving them attention. The result was that the children could only gain attention by demanding it in some inappropriate way (tantrums, etc.). Clare was instructed to withhold attention following annoying or aggravating behavior while offering more attention at other times.

The latter part of the session focused on increasing leisure activities. Clare initially argued that this was impossible because of her family commitments. After a discussion of the negative effects of her headaches on herself and her family, and the positive effects of increased hobbies and interests on her headaches, she relented and agreed to pursue this course of action. Various alternatives were considered and she said that she would join a health club or take up aerobics.

Her homework assignments were to put into practice the cognitive and behavioral approach to her problems with the children and to take steps toward increased hobbies (i.e., join a health club or an aerobics group).

SESSION 10

Review of the previous week suggested that Clare's attempts at changing her interactions with her children had met with some success. As had been anticipated in the office session, withholding attention for inappropriate behaviors led to a short-term increase in the behaviors as the children worked harder at gaining attention. Clare persisted, however, and later in the week the frequency of these behaviors began to decline.

Clare had not made much progress toward increasing leisure activities. She discovered that health club fees had increased, which was enough to dissuade her from joining. She was considering a course in computer programming, but the course did not begin until next term. Again, the advantages of increased hobbies were emphasized and she agreed to explore other options next week.

Some of the session was devoted to relaxation training using the relaxation by recall technique. Clare was also introduced to the method of differential relaxation. Cognitive training based on the maladaptive thoughts records constituted the final part of the session.

Homework assignments consisted of practicing relaxation by recall and differential relaxation in relatively undemanding situations. Clare was also asked to work on increasing her leisure activities.

SESSION 11

Jim was requested to attend this session as the main aim was to review the contingency management approach. His presence was also considered appropriate while reviewing progress in the child management area and efforts at increasing Clare's leisure activities.

Jim confirmed that Clare's attitude to the children had improved and she was responding to them more positively. He commented that she seemed to have gained confidence in her ability to cope with them.

With respect to leisure activities, Clare had arranged to go to the health club the following week. She had also arranged to audition for a singing role in a Gilbert and Sullivan musical and to join an acting company.

The contingency management procedure seemed to be working well, with decreases in Clare's tendency to request Jim to return from work to help her, increases in his offers of assistance, and Clare's beginning to attend more social occasions that she had previously avoided in case she got a headache. Both Clare and Jim thought the concept of contingency management was a "bit juvenile" and "false" but accepted it with good humor and could appreciate that it was having positive effects in breaking bad habits that had developed.

Homework assignments were for Jim to continue with the contingency management and for Clare to practice relaxation. Clare was also asked to continue with the child management strategies and follow up her leisure initiatives.

SESSION 12

In the review of events since the last appointment, Clare said that she had gotten very angry with her mother-in-law who had picked up her elder son from primary school, but instead of driving him home had made him walk home after getting upset with him. This incident was followed by a headache but was also a source of continuing tension. Discussion led to the decision that Clare would talk to her mother-in-law to try to resolve the friction. Role playing was used to rehearse how she would handle the situation.

The rest of the session was spent on relaxation training using recall and counting and imagery training following the sequence described in Chapter 10. Although the relaxation training continued to proceed smoothly, the imagery training did not go well as Clare rated the vividness and controllability of her images as low. Clare could not identify any imagery associated with her headaches and said that she did not use imagery to control headaches or other stressful situations.

Clare was asked to practice relaxation by recall and counting and differential relaxation in more demanding situations than previously. She was also requested to practice developing her imagery ability as outlined in Chapter 10.

SESSION 13

Clare's meeting with her mother-in-law resulted in a heated debate in which her mother-in-law told Clare that her children were badly behaved. Clare responded by giving her a lecture on the principles of child management. The argument seemed to clear the air between Clare and her mother-in-law. It also gave Clare the educational experience of defending her children against criticism which was a role reversal for her.

Having had no hobbies and interests for many years and showing resistance to developing any, Clare was rapidly moving toward an extensive range of leisure activities. After trying aerobics she decided that she wasn't an "exercise person." She had auditioned successfully for a musical show and joined an acting company. She had started a course in computer programming and was enjoying it. She had also become the coach for her eldest son's T-ball team.

Clare decided that she wanted to be a social worker. It was suggested to her that she might consider carrying out some voluntary work in the welfare field to see whether she was well suited to it before committing herself to extensive training.

Clare had practiced imagery training on most days since the last appointment but the ratings completed after practice indicated that she was still not achieving vivid or controllable images. Also, her practice diaries did not reveal any imagery associated with her headaches. In the session, another imagery exercise was completed with little success and it was decided to abandon this approach.

The session then focused on attention–diversion training following the procedure described in Chapter 10. Clare found the attentional exercise interesting and rated the degree of attentional control that she accomplished as quite high.

For homework, Clare was asked to practice developing control of attention. She was also asked to resume completing maladaptive thoughts records.

SESSION 14

Clare's practice at developing attentional control had gone well, with increased ratings following practice. An attentional exercise was completed to consolidate her progress with this technique. Relaxation training was then continued by using the counting procedure.

The rest of the session focused on cognitive training using the maladaptive thoughts records. The emphasis was on identifying underlying beliefs and countering them with verbal challenging and behavioral experiments.

As Clare's headaches had become infrequent, it was decided that the next session could probably be the final one. Clare was given copies of the BDI and STAI to complete the following morning and return by mail so that they could be scored prior to the next appointment. Homework consisted of applying attention–diversion strategies to any headaches that occurred. Also, Clare was asked to practice relaxation by counting and differential relaxation in demanding situations.

SESSION 15

Jim attended this session. Inspection of the records of practicing attention–diversion techniques indicated that Clare had experienced two headaches in the 2 weeks since her last appointment. She had responded to both first by relaxation and then using attention–diversion strategies. She particularly liked focusing attention on features of the environment as a cognitive coping strategy. Neither headache went above an intensity rating of 2, and they were of short duration (just under an hour and 2 hours).

The session then focused on review of progress. Clare said that she was only experiencing an occasional headache and so had dispensed with using medication. Both she and Jim thought that her relationship with the children had improved. She had a more positive image of them. Clare's hobbies and interests had increased dramatically. In fact, Jim thought that she had gone "a bit overboard." They both accepted that this was a reaction against her previous pain-dominated life-style and that she would progress toward a more intermediary course. Jim considered that Clare had become more relaxed and less irritable.

Consideration was given to whether any events or circumstances in the future could be identified that potentially would lead to relapse. It was noted that winter was approaching which had been associated with more headaches in the past. The most likely explanations of this association were that Clare did more cooking in winter and the children spent more time indoors. Clare felt confident that she could now cope with the children adequately and Jim was helping more with household activities, including cooking, so she believed that these conditions were manageable.

Another potentially problematic event was moving, as they had decided to build a larger home. Discussion focused on reducing the demands associated with these events (e.g., arranging for a moving company to pack and move their household effects rather than doing it themselves) and use of relaxation and cognitive coping skills to maintain low levels of arousal.

It was agreed that Clare would continue to practice relaxation on a daily basis at least for a few more weeks and would use relaxation, cognitive coping (i.e., identifying and challenging maladaptive thoughts), and attention–

diversion strategies to counter any headaches that occurred. No follow-up appointments were arranged because Clare and Jim felt confident that if problems arose they could solve them with the skills they had learned.

Treatment Outcome

Clare's headaches had steadily decreased over the 5 months of appointments in terms of frequency, duration, and intensity. The average intensity rating calculated from the daily cards dropped from .41 and .49 in the 2 weeks prior to treatment, to .03 and .01 in the final 2 weeks of treatment. Medication also decreased from an average daily pill count of 3.9 and 4.2 in the 2 weeks before treatment to no use of medication in the final 2 weeks of treatment.

Clare's score on the BDI dropped from the mildly depressed range pretreatment (14) to the normal range at the end of treatment (5). Her scores on the STAI shifted from the 75th percentile to the 57th percentile for state anxiety and from the 71st percentile to the 60th percentile for trait anxiety.

Case II: Frank

The patient, Frank, whose case was discussed in Chapter 8 and whose headaches were presented diagrammatically in Figure 8.2, was seen weekly for a total of 10 sessions. More sessions had been anticipated but Frank wished to discontinue at this point. Summarized below are the treatment plan, process of treatment, and treatment outcome.

Treatment Plan

The following techniques constituted the treatment plan:

1. Education
2. Relaxation training (autogenic training)
3. Cognitive training focusing on maladaptive thoughts and beliefs
4. Imagery training
5. Attention–diversion training
6. Modification of immediate antecedents
7. Modification of life-style factors aimed at increasing hobbies and interests
8. Training in time management and problem solving

Process of Treatment

PRIOR TO FIRST APPOINTMENT, AND SESSIONS 1 AND 2

The early contacts with Frank proceeded as for Clare and therefore involved administration of the Preassessment Patient Information Sheet immediately prior to the first appointment and an assessment interview following the format of the PAHQ across the first two sessions. Frank was instructed in use of the daily cards and asked to complete a BDI and STAI at the end of the first session. The results of these assessments are discussed in Chapter 8.

SESSION 3

This session was devoted to the educational component. Frank's wife, Hazel, had not been specifically invited to the session because the available information did not suggest that the behavior of the family was significantly involved in the etiology of the headaches, nor that the family was strongly affected by the headaches. Frank had been asked to tell his wife that she was welcome to attend if she wished to do so and would be invited to a later session to review progress. Hazel indicated that, under the circumstances, she would not attend until the later session.

The session followed the four-stage educational sequence outlined in Chapter 9 and concluded with instructions in how to complete the change and control cards. Frank was given a copy of the diagram of his headaches and asked to discuss it with Hazel.

SESSION 4

This session started with a discussion of Hazel's reactions to the diagram of Frank's headaches. He reported that she indicated that it summed up the situation very well. She had particularly emphasized the role of his low self-esteem.

The remainder of the session focused on relaxation training. Frank had attended a weekend workshop on stress management 14 months previously. This workshop seemed to involve mainly progressive relaxation and "positive thinking." Frank reported that he found the positive thinking approach useful but didn't like the progressive relaxation because he had difficulty releasing the tension he created. After some discussion, it was decided to use autogenic training rather than try progressive relaxation again.

Autogenic training proceeded by outlining the rationale and then using the first standard exercise of "heaviness." Observation of Frank and changes in relaxation ratings suggested that Frank was able to use the formula quite effectively.

The session concluded with instructions for home practice aided by an audiotape and recording details of the practice. Frank was also asked to continue with the change and control cards for one more week.

SESSION 5

Inspection of Frank's relaxation records indicated that he had practiced relaxation every day assiduously but had interpreted "at least once but ideally twice each day" as "once a day." The need for finding more time to practice relaxation was emphasized. Frank's ratings of relaxation indicated that he was getting good results when he did use the technique.

Autogenic training continued with the second standard exercise of "warmth." This was followed by introducing cognitive training focusing on maladaptive thoughts and beliefs. This approach seemed appropriate for the usual three areas of application: stress and negative affect as antecedents of headaches and cognitive reactions to headaches mediating maladaptive affective and behavioral responses such as yelling at the family (see Chapter 11). The approach also seemed relevant to predisposing factors as these factors would manifest themselves in thoughts and underlying beliefs: (1) Type A, thoughts and beliefs related to anger; (2) perfectionism, thoughts, and beliefs related to high standards; and (3) low self-esteem and guilt, thoughts, and beliefs related to self-criticism and self-denigration.

The rationale of cognitive training was discussed and the completed change and control cards were used to provide examples of Frank's maladaptive thoughts. As homework, Frank was asked to complete the maladaptive thoughts records and to practice relaxation using the warmth formula with the aid of a new audiotape.

SESSION 6

Frank had practiced relaxation twice a day on most days since the last appointment. He had completed some maladaptive thoughts records quite satisfactorily except for a tendency to use a rather limited range of rational responses. Also, he hadn't set up any behavioral experiments. The first part of the session was spent going back through verbal challenging, emphasizing the methods that he had not used and discussing behavioral experiments that would have been appropriate.

The second part of the session focused on modifying the immediate antecedents of headaches. As noted in Chapter 8, the two main themes in the antecedents were stress and negative affect and visual factors. Frank had tried to counter the visual problems via altering the physical environment (i.e., glasses, alternative computer screens, lighting) but had not considered a behavioral approach. Because a headache tended to develop after approximately 30 minutes of viewing, Frank was encouraged to experiment with different schedules such as working on the computer for 20 to 30 minutes then taking a break for 5 to 10 minutes during which time he did something else. He argued initially that this was not possible, but after further discussion agreed that he might be able to rearrange his commitments in this way.

Loud noise was not a common precipitant and could probably be managed by more determined efforts to avoid its occurrence. With respect to cigarette smoke, both physical (e.g., use of a desk fan) and behavioral (e.g., use of assertive responses) strategies were discussed, with an emphasis on the latter. Frowning while concentrating was targeted as a behavior to be modified by developing relaxation skills.

Frank was asked to put into practice the strategies for reducing trigger factors, in particular, the change of habits for working on the computer. He was asked to continue with the maladaptive thoughts records, but to take a break from relaxation practice.

SESSION 7

Frank had tried to insert breaks into his work on the computer but to no avail. There seemed to be a number of problems with his efforts, however. For example, he didn't plan his work around such a schedule but instead would work on the computer, suddenly remember he should take a break, and reluctantly do so. He found the breaks disruptive and frustrating, which may have canceled out any beneficial effects. It was agreed that he would try again with more forward planning.

The rest of the session focused on setting factors. As noted in Chapter 8, he had been a keen sportsman, but his recreational activities had fallen away to an occasional game of tennis. Discussion took place with respect to appropriate ways of increasing exercise and leisure activities. Given that one of the factors inhibiting him in this area was guilt related to the fact that Hazel didn't devote any time to hobbies and interests, recreational activities that could involve her, and that she would enjoy, were considered a priority. It was agreed that he would take up ballroom dancing as he had some interest in doing so and Hazel was very keen on it. It was also agreed that he would play tennis more regularly (at least once a week), and start jogging two or three times a week.

Some time was then spent on training in time management and problem solving. The former was deemed appropriate because of Frank's Type A approach to life characterized by a feeling of time pressure ("hurry sickness").

Frank started treatment feeling somewhat overwhelmed by his commitments and the treatment program was calling for him to invest significant amounts of time in homework assignments and to develop new hobbies and interests.

Problem solving was considered a useful technique for him to resolve some of the problems he was experiencing at work and at home. One example was provided by his son's Marfan's syndrome. The distinction between emotion-focused and problem-focused forms of coping was discussed (Lazarus & Folkman, 1984) and practical steps toward reducing his worries were considered. Questioning revealed that the son was overdue for a medical examination which Frank and Hazel had not arranged because of their fears. It was agreed that their worries were multiplying in the absence of medical advice and so they should set up an appointment.

Frank was asked to put into practice the life-style techniques discussed in the session and to continue the maladaptive thoughts records.

SESSION 8

Review of the week's activities indicated that Frank had followed through on the increased activities plan. He and Hazel had attended their first ballroom dancing session and enjoyed it. Frank had played tennis on the weekend and Hazel had accompanied him. He had jogged on two occasions, once on his own and once with his son. He was pleasantly surprised at the level of fitness these activities revealed.

Frank had applied problem-solving approaches to some of his problems with time pressure. He had accepted his father's offer to take over mowing Frank's grass. Also, housekeeping had been a source of friction between Frank and Hazel because her efforts at keeping the family home clean and tidy did not match up to Frank's exacting standards. They agreed to employ someone to carry out these activities for them.

The next part of the session was devoted to autogenic training using the third standard formula of "cardiac regulation." The final part of the session focused on cognitive training. The maladaptive thoughts records were used to identify underlying beliefs.

Homework consisted of relaxation practice using a new audiotape and use of the maladaptive thoughts records with particular emphasis on challenging maladaptive beliefs and designing behavioral experiments to test the beliefs.

SESSION 9

At the start of this session, Frank indicated that he would like to discontinue treatment at this stage since his headaches had decreased substantially and he now knew what he had to do to get on top of his headache problem. This decision was discouraged since he was still experiencing some headaches and the treatment plan had not been completed, but he was keen to try on his own. Agreement was reached that one more session would be scheduled, and Hazel would be asked to attend that session.

The session proceeded with autogenic training using the fourth standard exercise of "respiration." The remainder of the session focused on imagery training according to the sequence described in Chapter 10. Imagery training followed well from autogenic training given the emphasis in both on visualization. Frank rated the images he produced as both vivid and controllable. He could not identify any images associated with his headaches but said he did imagine himself in pleasant situations as a stress coping strategy.

Homework consisted of relaxation practice using the respiration formula and practice at developing imagery ability. As the imagery exercises had gone well in the office session and only one more appointment was planned, Frank was also asked to practice using imagery as a pain-coping strategy. That is, both phases of imagery home practice were started simultaneously. Finally, Frank was given a BDI to complete and return by post before the final session.

SESSION 10

Only Frank was present in the first part of this session as the initial aim was to review the previous week's homework assignments and to conclude the autogenic training. Home practice of imagery had gone well and Frank had used imagery strategies to counter headaches on two occasions. He found transformative imagery particularly helpful. Ratings of imagery vividness and controllability were consistently high.

Autogenic training concluded with the fifth standard exercise of "abdominal warmth." As with all the previous formulae, Frank was able to use it to achieve a significant increase in relaxation.

At this stage, Hazel was invited into the session to review progress. She said that she had noticed many positive changes in Frank including an improvement in his self-esteem, although she felt that he would benefit from further changes in this area. She volunteered that be approached life in a more relaxed manner but seemed to have to "work at it" rather than have it come naturally. They were both spending more time on recreational activities and enjoying doing so. Frank had recently added golf to the ballroom dancing, tennis, and jogging. Frank believed that organizing his computer work to include regular breaks had helped his headaches but not solved the problem completely.

Events and circumstances that could lead to relapse were considered. The main danger identified was the possibility of Frank's company being sold, leaving him without a job. His self-confidence had increased to the point, however, that he believed he could make a success of starting his own business as a construction programmer.

Frank felt that all the pain management strategies he had learned— relaxation, cognitive coping, and imagery—were useful and that he would continue to use them when needed.

Treatment Outcome

Average headache intensity ratings calculated from the daily cards indicated Frank's headaches had decreased from .72 and .64 in the 2 weeks before treatment to .25 and .21 in the final 2 weeks of treatment. This represented a reduction in headache activity of 66.2%. Medication usage decreased from an average consumption of three to four pills each day prior to treatment to an average consumption of less than one a day at the end of treatment.

Frank's score on the BDI dropped from the moderately depressed range before treatment (21) to the mildly depressed range at the end of treatment (11).

APPENDIX 1

Headache Classification System (HCC, 1988)

1. Migraine
    1.1 Migraine without aura
    1.2 Migraine with aura
        1.2.1 Migraine with typical aura
        1.2.2 Migraine with prolonged aura
        1.2.3 Familial hemiplegic migraine
        1.2.4 Basilar migraine
        1.2.5 Migraine aura without headache
        1.2.6 Migraine with acute onset aura
    1.3 Ophthalmoplegic migraine
    1.4 Retinal migraine
    1.5 Childhood periodic syndromes that may be precursors to or associated with migraine
        1.5.1 Benign paroxysmal vertigo of childhood
        1.5.2 Alternating hemiplegia of childhood
    1.6 Complications of migraine
        1.6.1 Status migrainosus
        1.6.1 Migrainous infarction
    1.7 Migrainous disorder not fulfilling above criteria
2. Tension-type headache
    2.1 Episodic tension-type headache
        2.1.1 Episodic tension-type headache associated with disorder of pericranial muscles
        2.1.2 Episodic tension-type headache unassociated with disorder of pericranial muscles
    2.2 Chronic tension-type headache
        2.2.1 Chronic tension-type headache associated with disorder of pericranial muscles

      2.2.2 Chronic tension-type headache unassociated with disorder of peri-cranial muscles

    2.3 Headache of the tension-type not fulfilling above criteria

3. Cluster headache and chronic paroxysmal hemicrania
4. Miscellaneous headaches unassociated with structural lesion
5. Headache associated with head trauma
6. Headache associated with vascular disorders
7. Headache associated with nonvascular intracranial disorder
8. Headache associated with substances or their withdrawal
9. Headache associated with noncephalic infection
10. Headache associated with metabolic disorder
11. Headache or facial pain associated with disorder of cranium, neck, eyes, ears, nose, sinuses, teeth, mouth, or other facial or cranial structures
12. Cranial neuralgias, nerve trunk pain, and deafferentation pain
13. Headache not classifiable

Note. Subcategories are not shown for categories 3–13.

APPENDIX 2

Diagnostic Guidelines for Use with the Psychological Assessment of Headache Questionnaire

1.1 Migraine without aura

Description: Idiopathic, recurring headache disorder manifesting in attacks lasting 4–72 hours. Typical characteristics of headache are unilateral location, pulsating quality, moderate or severe intensity, aggravation by routine physical activity, and association with nausea, photo-, and phonophobia (HCC, 1988, p. 19).

At least five attacks fulfilling the following criteria:
1. R3 to Q6.
2. At least two of the following: R1 to Q2, R1 to Q1, R2 or R3 to Q7, and R1 to Q9.
3. R1 to Q10.1 and/or R1 to Q10.2, or R1 to Q10.3 and R1 to Q10.4.

1.2.1 Migraine with typical aura

Description: Migraine with an aura consisting of homonymous visual disturbances, hemiparesis or dysphasia, or combinations thereof. Gradual development, duration under 1 hour, and complete reversibility characterize the aura which is associated with headache (HCC, 1988, p. 22).

At least two attacks fulfilling the following criteria:
1. R1 to Q12.
2. R1 to Q13
3. R1 to Q14.
4. R1 to Q15.
Also, R1 to either Q11.1, Q11.2, Q11.3 or Q11.4.

2.1 Episodic tension-type headache

Description: Recurrent episodes of headache lasting minutes to days. The pain is typically pressing/tightening in quality, of mild or moderate intensity, bilateral in location, and does not worsen with routine physical activity. Nausea is absent, but photophobia or phonophobia may be present (HCC, 1988, p. 29).

At least 10 previous headache episodes fulfilling the following criteria:
1. R1 to Q8.
2. R2 or R3 or R4 to Q6.
3. At least two of the following: R2 to Q1; R1 or R2 to Q7; R2 to Q2; and R2 to Q9.
4. R2 to Q10.1 and R2 to Q10.2; and R2 to Q10.3 or R2 to Q10.4.

2.2 Chronic tension-type headache
Description: Headache present for at least 15 days a month during at least 6 months. The headache is usually pressing/tightening in quality, mild or moderate in severity, bilateral, and does not worsen with routine physical activity. Nausea, photophobia, or phonophobia may occur (HCC, 1988, p. 31).

Headaches present for at least 6 months fulfilling the following criteria:
1. R2 to Q8.
2. At least two of the following: R2 to Q1, R1 or R2 to Q7, R2 to Q2, and R2 to Q9.
3. R2 to Q10.2 and no more than one of the following: R1 to Q10.1, R1 to Q10.3, R1 to Q10.4.

2.3 Headache of the tension-type not fulfilling above criteria
Description: Headache that is believed to be a form of tension-type headache but does not quite meet the operational diagnostic criteria for any of the forms of tension-type headache (HCC, 1988, p. 32)..

Headaches fulfilling the following criteria:
1. Fulfills all but one criterion for one or more forms of tension-type headache.
2. Does not fulfil criteria for migraine without aura.

Note. The PAHQ appears in full in Appendix 4. In the guidelines, Q = Question and R = Response, so that question 3 on the PAHQ, for example, is referred to as Q3 and the response numbered 1 as R1.

APPENDIX 3

Preassessment Patient Information Sheet

Assessment and Treatment of Headaches from a Psychological Perspective

Assessment of headaches from a psychological viewpoint is aimed at achieving a better understanding of headaches. Key questions include: Why do the headaches occur or get worse at one time rather than another? and Why is the patient particularly vulnerable to headaches currently? Assessment usually involves a couple of interviews and patients keeping records of their headaches on cards.

Assessment particularly focuses on three areas. First, what are the factors that precipitate or aggravate headaches (e.g., stress, eyestrain, certain foods)? Second, what are the life-style factors that make the patient liable to suffer from headaches? For example, if headaches are precipitated or aggravated by stress, what are the main sources of stress for the patient? The third important area is to investigate the responses of patients to their headaches and the reactions of their families. Patients often respond to headaches in ways that are understandable (e.g., becoming angry, tense, and depressed or being irritable with their families), but can result in their getting locked into headache–stress–headache vicious cycles.

Treatment is based on the results of the assessment and varies according to the specific nature of the patient's headaches. The starting point is an educational component in which headaches are discussed generally, followed by consideration of the particular causes of the patient's headaches. Treatment then proceeds at three main levels. The first involves training in pain management skills that are designed to prevent headaches developing or to reduce their intensity and duration if they do occur. Pain management techniques include relaxation training, use of imagery to combat pain, attention–diversion training, and control of thoughts as a method of controlling feelings and pain. A second level of treatment involves changing the life-style factors that encourage headaches. If, for example, headaches involve stress, treatment would attempt to eliminate the stressors, or help patients cope with the stressors better. The third level of treatment consists of helping patients and their families to respond to headaches in the most appropriate ways (ie., ways that minimize headaches rather than aggravate them).

Treatment usually takes 10 to 15 sessions to complete. Treatment sessions are supplemented by patients practicing developing skills at home with the help of written and taperecorded instructions. Results of treatment vary and are difficult to predict, but most headache patients show some improvement and many are able to reduce their headaches to "normal" levels (i.e., occasional headaches as experienced by most of the population).

APPENDIX 4

Psychological Assessment of Headache Questionnaire (PAHQ)

Part I: Personal and Social History

Name: _____

Address: _____

_____

Telephone number: (h) _____   (w) _____

(A) Date of birth: _____   Sex: M/F

Marital status: S/M/D/W/other _____

Current occupation: Past occupation(s):

Nationality: Place of birth:

Religion: Preferred hand:

Highest educational level:

Hobbies and interests:

Cigarette smoking:

Alcohol consumption:

Contraceptive pill (type, duration):

(A) History of major illnesses and injuries:

Note. Questions denoted by "A" (for Alert) provide information with respect to danger signs and symptoms. Questions denoted by "D" (for Diagnosis) provide information for making a diagnosis based on the IHS classification system.

Current health problems other than headaches:

Other problems (social, financial, etc.):

Current treatments for other health problems:

Type of accommodation (owner occupier/rented, house/unit):

Cohabitants:

Date(s) of marriage:

Date(s) of divorce:

Date(s) of death of spouse/partner:

Spouse/partner's	name:	age:	occupation:
Father's	name:	age:	occupation:
Mother's	name:	age:	occupation:
Child's 1	name:	age:	occupation:
Child's 2	name:	age:	occupation:
Child's 3	name:	age:	occupation:
Child's 4	name:	age:	occupation:
Brother's 1	name:	age:	occupation:
Brother's 2	name:	age:	occupation:
Sister's 1	name:	age:	occupation:
Sister's 2	name:	age:	occupation:

(A) Changes in personality or behavior:

(A) Changes in memory or intellectual functioning:

(A) Family history of . . .

      Cerebral aneurysm or other vascular anomalies:

      Polycystic kidneys:

Other information:

Part II: Headaches

Can you identify more than one type of headache, each of which constitutes a
significant problem?

Yes	No
1	2

Complete Part II for each type of headache.

Section A: Headaches and Associated Symptoms

(D) 1. How do the headaches feel?

	Pressing/	
Pulsating	tightening	Other
1	2	3

If "other," specify _____

(A,D) 2. Are the headaches. . . .

Unilateral	Bilateral
1	2

(A) 3. If unilateral, have they always been on the same side?

Yes	No
1	2

4. Where is the pain?

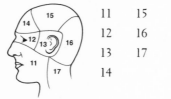

11	15	21	25
12	16	22	26
13	17	23	27
14		24	

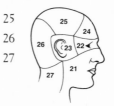

(A) 5. Are the headaches constant and unremitting?

Yes	No
1	2

(D) 6. How long do the headaches last (untreated or unsuccessfully treated)?

Less than 30 min	30 min–4 hr	4 hr–72 hr	72 hr–7 days	More than 7 days
1	2	3	4	5

(D) 7. How intense are the headaches?

Mild	Moderate	Severe
1	2	3

(D) 8. Is the average headache frequency . . .

Less than 15 days per month	15 days per month or more
1	2

(D) 9. Are the headaches aggravated by walking stairs or similar routine physical activity?

Yes	No
1	2

(A,D) 10. Are the headaches accompanied by . . .

	Yes	No
10.1 Nausea	1	2
10.2 Vomiting	1	2
10.3 Photophobia	1	2
10.4 Phonophobia	1	2

(A,D) 11. Have the following aura symptoms preceded or accompanied at least two headaches?

	Yes	No
11.1 Homonymous visual disturbance	1	2
11.2 Unilateral paresthesias and/or numbness	1	2
11.3 Unilateral weakness	1	2
11.4 Aphasia or unclassifiable speech difficulty	1	2
11.5 Visual symptoms in both the temporal and nasal fields of both eyes	1	2
11.6 Dysarthria	1	2

	Yes	No
11.7 Vertigo	1	2
11.8 Tinnitus	1	2
11.9 Decreased hearing	1	2
11.10 Double vision	1	2
11.11 Ataxia	1	2
11.12 Bilateral paresthesias	1	2
11.13 Bilateral pareses	1	2
11.14 Decreased level of consciousness	1	2
11.15 Monocular scotoma or blindness	1	2

(D) 12. Based on the answers to question 11 above, are there one or more fully reversible aura symptoms indicating focal cerebral cortical and/or brain stem dysfunction?

Yes   No
1   2

(D) 13. Does at least one aura symptom develop gradually over more than 4 minutes or, 2 or more symptoms occur in succession?

Yes   No
1   2

(D) 14. Does no aura symptom last more than 60 minutes? (If more than one aura symptom is present, accepted duration is proportionally increased.)

Yes   No
1   2

(D) 15. Does the headache follow the aura with a free interval of less than 60 minutes? (It may also begin before or simultaneously with the aura.)

Yes   No
1   2

Section B: Functional Analysis

(A) 16. Are there any cycles in headaches?

16.1 Daily _____

16.2 Weekly _____

16.3 Monthly _____

16.4 Yearly _____

17. Do headaches ever . . .

	Never	Sometimes	Always
Delay sleep onset	1	2	3
Result in waking	1	2	3

If they sometimes result in waking what do you do: _____

_____

Does it lead to others waking?

	Never	Sometimes	Always
	1	2	3

If so, who: _____

What do they do: _____

IMMEDIATE ANTECEDENTS OF HEADACHE CHANGE

18. Do you know when a headache is coming on?

	Never	Sometimes	Always
	1	2	3

If you sometimes know, how: _____

19. What factors precipitate or aggravate headaches?

		Never	Rarely	Some-times	Usually	Always
19.1	Food	1	2	3	4	5
19.2	Hunger	1	2	3	4	5
19.3	Alcohol	1	2	3	4	5
19.4	Smoking	1	2	3	4	5
19.5	Exercise	1	2	3	4	5
19.6	Sexual activity	1	2	3	4	5

		Never	Rarely	Some-times	Usually	Always
19.7	Fatigue	1	2	3	4	5
19.8	Frowning	1	2	3	4	5
19.9	Jaw clenching	1	2	3	4	5
19.10	Neck movements	1	2	3	4	5
19.11	Coughing	1	2	3	4	5
19.12	Sneezing	1	2	3	4	5
19.13	Stress	1	2	3	4	5
19.14	Relaxation	1	2	3	4	5
19.15	Anxiety	1	2	3	4	5
19.16	Depression	1	2	3	4	5
19.17	Anger	1	2	3	4	5
19.18	Flicker	1	2	3	4	5
19.19	Glare	1	2	3	4	5
19.20	Eyestrain	1	2	3	4	5
19.21	Noise	1	2	3	4	5
19.22	Humidity	1	2	3	4	5
19.23	High temperature	1	2	3	4	5
19.24	Low temperature	1	2	3	4	5
19.25	Pollen count	1	2	3	4	5
19.26	Other _____	1	2	3	4	5

20. What factors relieve a headache?

		Never	Rarely	Some-times	Usually	Always
20.1	Drugs	1	2	3	4	5
20.2	Rest	1	2	3	4	5
20.3	Massage	1	2	3	4	5
20.4	Hot bath/shower	1	2	3	4	5
20.1	Alcohol	1	2	3	4	5
20.1	Other _____	1	2	3	4	5

IMMEDIATE CONSEQUENCES OF HEADACHE CHANGE

21. When a headache begins or gets worse. . . .

    21.1 What do you do?

		Never	Rarely	Some-times	Usually	Always
21.1.1	Stop what you are doing	1	2	3	4	5
21.1.2	Sit down	1	2	3	4	5
21.1.3	Lie down	1	2	3	4	5
21.1.4	Shower/bath	1	2	3	4	5
21.1.5	Take medication	1	2	3	4	5
21.1.6	Eat	1	2	3	4	5
21.1.7	Drink	1	2	3	4	5
21.1.8	Try distracting yourself	1	2	3	4	5
21.1.9	Try relaxing	1	2	3	4	5
21.1.10	Other _____	1	2	3	4	5

21.2 Do others know when you have a headache?

Never	Rarely	Some-times	Usually	Always
1	2	3	4	5

If so, who knows: _____

How do they know: _____

21.3 What do others do?

		Never	Rarely	Some-times	Usually	Always
21.3.1	Massage	1	2	3	4	5
21.3.2	Sympathize	1	2	3	4	5
21.3.3	Ignore	1	2	3	4	5
21.3.4	Complain	1	2	3	4	5
21.3.5	Get medication	1	2	3	4	5
21.3.6	Get food	1	2	3	4	5

		Never	Rarely	Some-times	Usually	Always
21.3.7	Get drink	1	2	3	4	5
21.3.8	Encourage you to stop what you are doing	1	2	3	4	5
21.3.9	Encourage you to sit down	1	2	3	4	5
21.3.10	Encourage you to lie down	1	2	3	4	5
21.3.11	Encourage you to keep going	1	2	3	4	5
21.3.12	Other _____	1	2	3	4	5

21.4 What thoughts do you have? _____

_____

21.5 What imagery occurs? _____

_____

21.6 How do you feel (checklist)? _____

_____

22. When a headache diminishes or ends. . . .

21.1 What do you do:

If you rest *during* a headache

Do you continue resting after

Never	Sometimes	Always
1	2	3

If you do continue resting, for how long _____

If you do not continue resting, do you return to previous or equivalent activity _____

Do you engage in easier tasks _____

22.2 Do others know when your headache ends?

	Never	Sometimes	Always
	1	2	3

If so, who knows: _____

How do they know: _____

22.3 What do others do?

	Never	Sometimes	Always
Encourage you to take it easy	1	2	3
Encourage you to get on	1	2	3
Other _____	1	2	3

22.4 What thoughts do you have? _____

_____

22.5 What imagery occurs? _____

_____

22.6 How do you feel (checklist)? _____

_____

LONG-TERM CONSEQUENCES OF HEADACHES

23.1 What effect does the headache problem have on. . . .

You _____

Your work _____

(Average days off work in a year resulting from headaches) _____

Your social/recreational activities _____

Other _____

Your partner _____

Anyone else _____

23.2 If you did not have a headache problem what would. . . .

You do _____

Your partner do _____

Anyone else do _____

HISTORY OF HEADACHES

(A) 24.1 When did headaches begin?

Day _____ Month _____ Year _____

24.2 Was the onset of the headaches . . .

Sudden	Gradual
1	2

(A) 24.3 Can you identify any event or circumstance that you think may have contributed to headaches beginning?

Yes	Possibly	No
1	2	3

If "possibly"/"yes" were the circumstances. . . .

Stressful events _____

Head or neck trauma _____

Menarche _____

Oral contraceptive _____

Pregnancy _____

Conditions of exertion such as lifting, during sexual intercourse, or during a heated argument _____

Other _____

(A) 24.4 Over time have they become?

Much higher frequency	Higher frequency	Same frequency	Lower frequency	Much lower frequency
1	2	3	4	5

Much higher intensity	Higher intensity	Same intensity	Lower intensity	Much lower intensity
1	2	3	4	5

Much longer duration	Longer duration	Same duration	Shorter duration	Much shorter duration
1	2	3	4	5

24.5 Were there any periods in which the headaches significantly diminished or disappeared?

Yes   No
1   2

If "yes," dates: _____
Circumstances: _____

24.6 Were there any periods in which the headaches significantly worsened?

Yes   No
1   2

If "yes," dates: _____
Circumstances: _____

RELATIVES AND CLOSE FRIENDS WITH HEADACHES

25. Have any of the following a significant headache problem? (Enter Y, yes; N, no; D, don't know.)

	Regular headaches	Received medical treatment for headaches	Additional information
Paternal grandfather			
Paternal grandmother			
Maternal grandfather			
Maternal grandmother			
Father			
Mother			
Partner/spouse			
Child 1 _____			
Child 2 _____			
Child 3 _____			
Child 4 _____			
Brother 1 _____			
Brother 2 _____			
Sister 1 _____			

	Regular headaches	Received medical treatment for headaches	Additional information
Sister 2	_____		
Other relatives	_____		
Close friends	_____		

Section C: Assessment and Treatment History

26. Have you had any investigations or tests for headaches?

    CAT scan   Date _____

    Spinal puncture   Date _____

    Radioisotope scan   Date _____

    Myelography   Date _____

    Ventriculography   Date _____

    Angiography   Date _____

    Pneumoencephalography   Date _____

    Other _____   Date _____

27. Have you been to see any specialists about headaches?

    Neurologist   Date _____

    General practitioner   Date _____

    Other medical   Date _____

    Psychologist   Date _____

    Chiropractor/osteopath   Date _____

    Physiotherapist   Date _____

    Other _____   Date _____

28. Past treatments for headaches include:

               Treatment A   Treatment B

Type _____

Dates _____

Effects* _____

               Treatment C   Treatment D

Type _____

Dates _____

Effects* _____

29. Current treatments for headaches include:

               Treatment A   Treatment B

Type _____

Dates _____

Effects* _____

*Include in the "effects" box, a rating for each treatment on the following scale:

Very effective	Moderately effective	Slightly effective	Not at all effective
1	2	3	4

References

Adams, H. E. (1985). Case formulations of chronic headaches. In I. D. Turkat (Ed.), *Behavioral case formulations* (pp. 93–110). New York: Plenum Press.

Ad Hoc Committee. (1962). Classification of headache. *Journal of American Medical Association, 179,* 717–718.

Ahles, T. A., & Martin, J. B. (1989). The relationship of electromyographic and vasomotor activity to MMPI subgroups in chronic headache patients: The use of the original and contemporary MMPI norms. *Headache, 29,* 584–587.

Ahles, T. A., Martin, J. B., Gaulier, B., Cassens, H. L., Andres, M. L., & Shariff, M. (1988). Electromyographic and vasomotor activity in tension, migraine, and combined headache patients: The influence of postural variation. *Behaviour Research and Therapy, 26,* 519–525.

Alexander, A. B. (1975). An experimental test of assumptions relating to the use of electromygraphic feedback as a general relaxation training technique. *Psychophyisology, 12,* 656–662.

Allan, W. (1930). The inheritance of migraine. *Archives of Internal Medicine, 42,* 590–599.

Allen, R. A., & Weinmann, R. L. (1982). The McGill–Melzack Pain Questionnaire in the diagnosis of headache. *Headache, 22,* 20–29.

Al-Rajeh, S., Bademosi, O., Ismail, H., & Awada, A. (1990). Headache syndromes in the Eastern Province of Saudi Arabia. *Headache, 30,* 359–362.

Anciano, D. (1986). The pain behaviour checklist: Factor analysis and validation. *British Journal of Clinical Psychology, 25,* 301–302.

Anderson, C. D., & Franks, R. D. (1981). Migraine and tension headache: Is there a physiological difference? *Headache, 21,* 63–71.

Anderson, C. D., Stoyva, J. M., & Vaughn, L. J. (1982). A test of delayed recovery following stressful stimulation in four psychosomatic disorders. *Journal of Psychosomatic Research, 26,* 571–580.

Anderson, J. A. D., Basker, M. A., & Dalton, R. (1975). Migraine and hypnotherapy. *International Journal of Clinical and Experimental Hypnosis, 23,* 48–58.

Anderson, N. B., Lawrence, P. S., & Olson, T. W. (1981). Within-subject analysis of autogenic training and cognitive coping training in the treatment of tension headache pain. *Journal of Behavior Therapy and Experimental Psychiatry, 12,* 219–223.

Andrasik, F., Blanchard, E. B., Ahles, T., Pallmeyer, T., & Barron, K. D. (1981). Assessing the reactive as well as the sensory component of headache pain. *Headache, 21,* 218–221.

Andrasik, F., Blanchard, E. B., Arena, J. E., Saunders, N. L., & Barron, K. D. (1982). Psychophysiology of recurrent headache: Methodological issues and new empirical findings. *Behavior Therapy, 13,* 407–429.

Andrasik, F., Blanchard, E. B., Arena, J. G., Teders, S. J., & Rodichok, L. D. (1982). Cross validation of the Kudrow-Sutkus MMPI classification system for diagnosing headache type. *Headache, 22,* 2–5.

Andrasik, F., Blanchard, E. B., Arena, J. G., Teders, S. J., Teevan, R. C., & Rodichok, L. D. (1982). Psychological functioning in headache sufferers. *Psychosomatic Medicine, 44,* 171–182.

Andrasik, F., Blanchard, E. B., Neff, D. F., & Rodichok, L. D. (1984). Biofeedback and relaxation training for chronic headache: A controlled comparison of booster treatments and regular contacts for long-term maintenance. *Journal of Consulting and Clinical Psychology, 52,* 609–615.

Andrasik, F., & Holroyd, K. A. (1980a). A test of specific and nonspecific effects in the biofeedback treatment of tension headache. *Journal of Consulting and Clinical Psychology, 48,* 575–586.

Andrasik, F., & Holroyd, K. A. (1980b). Physiologic and self-report comparisons between tension headache sufferers and nonheadache controls. *Journal of Behavioral Assessment, 2,* 135–141.

Andrasik, F., & Holroyd, K. A. (1980c). Reliability and concurrent validity of headache questionnaire data. *Headache, 20,* 44–46.

Andrasik, F., Holroyd, K. A., & Abell, T. (1979). Prevalence of headache within a college student population: A preliminary analysis. *Headache, 19,* 384–387.

Andreychuk, T., & Skriver, C. (1975). Hypnosis and biofeedback in the treatment of migraine headache. *International Journal of Clinical and Experimental Hypnosis, 23,* 172–183.

Appelbaum, K. A., Blanchard, E. B., Nicholson, N. L., Radnitz, C., Kirsch, C., Michultka, D., Attanasio, V., Andrasik, F., & Dentinger, M. P. (1990). Controlled evaluation of the addition of cognitive strategies to a home-based relaxation protocol for tension headache. *Behavior Therapy, 21,* 293–303.

Appelbaum, K. A., Radnitz, C. L., Blanchard, E. B., & Prins, A. (1988). The pain behavior questionnaire (PBQ): A global report of pain behavior in chronic headaches. *Headache, 28,* 53–58.

Appenzeller, O., Davison, K., & Marshall, J. (1963). Reflex vasomotor abnormalities in the hands of migrainous subjects. *Journal of Neurology, Neurosurgery and Psychiatry, 26,* 447–450.

Arena, J. G., Andrasik, F., & Blanchard, E. B. (1985). The role of personality in the etiology of chronic headache. *Headache, 25,* 296–301.

Arena, J. G., Blanchard, E. B., & Andrasik, F. (1984). The role of affect in the etiology of chronic headache. *Journal of Psychosomatic Research, 28,* 79–86.

Arena, J. G., Blanchard, E. B., Andrasik, F., & Appelbaum, K. (1986). Obsessions and compulsions in three kinds of headache sufferers: Analysis of the Maudsley questionnaire. *Behaviour Research and Therapy, 24,* 127–132.

Arena, J. G., Blanchard, E. B., Andrasik, F., Appelbaum, K., & Myers, P. E. (1985). Psychophysiological comparisons of three kinds of headache subjects during and between headache states: Analysis of post-stress adaptation periods. *Journal of Psychosomatic Research, 29,* 427–441.

Arena, J. G., Blanchard, E. B., Andrasik, F., Cotch, P. A., & Myers, P. E. (1983). Reliability of psychophysiological assessment. *Behaviour Research and Therapy, 21,* 447–460.

Arena, J. G., Blanchard, E. B., Andrasik, F., & Dudek, B. C. (1982). The headache symptom questionnaire: Discriminant classificatory ability and headache syndromes suggested by a factor analysis. *Journal of Behavioral Assessment, 4,* 55–69.

Arena, J. G., Hannah, S. L., Bruno, G. M., & Meador, K. J. (1991). Electromyographic biofeedback training for tension headache in the elderly: A prospective study. *Biofeedback and Self-Regulation, 16,* 379–390.

Arena, J. G., Hightower, N. E., & Chong, G. C. (1988). Relaxation therapy for tension headache in the elderly: A prospective study. *Psychology and Aging, 3*, 96–98.

Askmark, H., Lundberg, P. O., & Olsson, S. (1989). Drug-related headache. *Headache, 29*, 441–444.

Attanasio, V., & Andrasik, F. (1987). Further examination of headache in the college student population. *Headache, 27*, 216–233.

Attanasio, V., Andrasik, F., & Blanchard, E. B. (1987). Cognitive therapy and relaxation training in muscle contraction headache: Efficacy and cost-effectiveness. *Headache, 27*, 254–260.

Bakal, D. A. (1982). *The psychobiology of chronic headache.* New York: Springer.

Bakal, D. A., Demjen, S., & Kaganov, J. A. (1981). Cognitive behavioral treatment of chronic headache. *Headache, 21*, 81–86.

Bakal, D. A., & Kaganov, J. A. (1976). A simple method for self-observation of headache frequency, intensity and location. *Headache, 16*, 123–124.

Bakal, D. A., & Kaganov, J. A. (1977). Muscle contraction and migraine headache: Psychophysiologic comparison. *Headache, 17*, 208–215.

Bakal, D. A., & Kaganov, J. A. (1979). Symptom characteristics of chronic and non-chronic headache sufferers. *Headache, 19*, 285–287.

Bana, D. S., Graham, J. R., & Spierings, E. L. H. (1988). Headache patients as they see themselves. *Headache, 28*, 403–408.

Bana, D. S., Leviton, A., Slack, W. V., Geer, D. E., & Graham, J. R. (1981). Use of a computerized data base in a headache clinic. *Headache, 21*, 72–74.

Bana, D. S., Leviton, A., Swidler, C., Slack, W., & Graham, J. R. (1980). A computer-based headache interview: Acceptance by patients and physicians. *Headache, 20*, 85–89.

Barlow, D. H. (1988). *Anxiety and its disorders: The nature and treatment of anxiety and panic.* New York: Guilford Press.

Barlow, D. H., Hayes, S. C., & Nelson, R. O. (1984). *The scientist practitioner: Research and accountability in clinical and educational settings.* New York: Pergamon Press.

Barnat, M. R., & Lake, A. E. (1983). Patient attitudes about headache. *Headache, 23*, 229–237.

Baumgartner, C., Wessely, P., Bingol, C., Maly, J., & Holzner, F. (1989). Long-term prognosis of analgesic withdrawal in patients with drug-induced headaches. *Headache, 29*, 510–514.

Beck, A. T., & Emery, G. (1985). *Anxiety disorders and phobias: A cognitive perspective.* New York: Basic Books.

Beck, A. T., Hollon, S. D., Young, J. E., Bedrosian, R. C., & Budenz, D. (1985). Treatment of depression with cognitive therapy and amitriptyline. *Archives of General Psychiatry, 42*, 142–148.

Beck, A. T., Rush, A. J., Shaw, B. F., & Emery, G. D. (1979). *Cognitive therapy of depression.* New York: Guilford Press.

Beck, A. T., Ward, C. H., Mendelsohn, M., Mock, J., & Erbaugh, J. (1961). An inventory for measuring depression. *Archives of General Psychiatry, 4*, 561–571.

Beecher, H. K. (1959). *Measurement of subjective response: Quantitative effects of drugs.* New York: Oxford University Press.

Benson, H., Klemchuk, H. P., & Graham, J. R. (1974). The usefulness of the relaxation response in the therapy of headache. *Headache, 14*, 49–52.

Benson, H., Malvea, B. P., & Graham, J. R. (1973). Physiologic correlates of meditation and their clinical effects in headache: An ongoing investigation. *Headache, 13*, 23–24.

Bergner, M., Bobbitt, R. A., Carter, W. B., & Gilson, B. S. (1981). The sickness impact profile: Development of and final version of a health status measure. *Medical Care, 19*, 787–805.

Bernstein, D. A., & Borkovec, T. D. (1973). *Progressive relaxation training: A manual for the helping professions.* Champaign, IL: Research Press.

Bild, R., & Adams, H. E. (1980). Modification of migraine headaches by cephalic blood volume pulse and EMG biofeedback. *Journal of Consulting and Clinical Psychology, 48*, 51–57.

Bille, B. S. (1962). Migraine in school children. *Acta Paediatrica Scandinavia, 51*(Suppl. 136), 1–151.

Bille, B. S. (1981). Migraine in childhood and its prognosis. *Cephalalgia, 1*, 71–75.

Blanchard, E. B. (1987). Long-term effects of behavioral treatment of chronic headache. *Behavior Therapy, 18*, 375–385.

Blanchard, E. B., & Andrasik, F. (1985). *Management of chronic headaches: A psychological approach.* New York: Pergamon Press.

Blanchard, E. B., Andrasik, F., Ahles, T. A., Teders, S. J., & O'Keefe, D. (1980). Migraine and tension headache: A meta-analytic review. *Behavior Therapy, 11*, 613–631.

Blanchard, E. B., Andrasik, F., Appelbaum, K. A., Evans, D. D., Jurish, S. E., Teders, S. J., Rodichok, L. D., & Barron, K. D. (1985). The efficacy and cost effectiveness of minimal therapist contact, nondrug treatments of chronic migraine and tension headache. *Headache, 25*, 214–220.

Blanchard, E. B., Andrasik, F., Appelbaum, K. A., Evans, D. D., Myers, P., & Barron, K. D. (1986). Three studies of the psychologic changes in chronic headache patients associated with biofeedback and relaxation therapies. *Psychosomatic Medicine, 48*, 73–83.

Blanchard, E. B., Andrasik, F., & Arena, J. G. (1984). Personality and chronic headache. *Progress in Experimental Personality Research, 13*, 303–360.

Blanchard, E. B., Andrasik, F., Arena, J. G., Neff, D. F., Jurish, S. E., Teders, S. J., Barron, K. D., & Rodichok, L. D. (1983). Nonpharmacologic treatment of chronic headache: Prediction of outcome. *Neurology, 33*, 1596–1603.

Blanchard, E. B., Andrasik, F., Arena, J. G., & Teders, S. J. (1982). Variation in meaning of pain descriptors for different headache types as revealed by psychophysical scaling. *Headache, 22*, 137–139.

Blanchard, E. B., Andrasik, F., Evans, D. D., & Hillhouse, J. (1985). Biofeedback and relaxation treatments for headache in the elderly: A caution and a challenge. *Biofeedback and Self-Regulation, 10*, 69–73.

Blanchard, E. B., Andrasik, F., Evans, D. D., Neff, D. F., Appelbaum, K. A., & Rodichok, L. D. (1985). Behavioral treatment of 250 chronic headache patients: A clinical replication series. *Behavior Therapy, 16*, 308–327.

Blanchard, E. B., Andrasik, F., Neff, D. F., Arena, J. G., Ahles, T. A., Jurish, S. E., Pallmeyer, T. P., Saunders, N. L., Teders, S. J., Barron, K. D., & Rodichok, L. D. (1982). Biofeedback and relaxation training with three kinds of headache: Treatment effects and their prediction. *Journal of Consulting and Clinical Psychology, 50*, 552–575.

Blanchard, E. B., Andrasik, F., Neff, D. F., Jurish, S. E., & O'Keefe, D. M. (1981). Social validation of the headache diary. *Behavior Therapy, 12*, 711–715.

Blanchard, E. B., Andrasik, F., Neff, D. F., Saunders, N. L., Arena, J. G., Pallmeyer, T. P., Teders, S. J., Jurish, S. E., & Rodichok, L. D. (1983). Four process studies in the behavioural treatment of chronic headache. *Behaviour Research and Therapy, 21*, 209–220.

Blanchard, E. B., Andrasik, F., Neff, D. F., Teders, S. J., Pallmeyer, T. P., Arena, J. G., Jurish, S. E., Saunders, N. L., Ahles, T. A., & Rodichok, L. D. (1982). Sequential comparisons of relaxation training and biofeedback in the treatment of three kinds of chronic headache or, the machines may be necessary some of time. *Behaviour Research and Therapy, 20*, 469–481.

Blanchard, E. B., Appelbaum, K. A., Guarnieri, P., Neff, D. F., Andrasik, F., Jaccard, J., & Barron, K. D. (1988). Two studies of the long-term follow-up of minimal therapist contact treatments of vascular and tension headache. *Journal of Consulting and Clinical Psychology, 56*, 427–432.

Blanchard, E. B., Appelbaum, K. A., Nicholson, N. L., Radnitz, C. L., Morill, B., Michultka, D., Kirsch, C., Hillhouse, J., & Dentinger, M. P. (1990). A controlled evaluation of the addition of cognitive therapy to a home-based biofeedback and relaxation treatment of vascular headache. *Headache, 30,* 371–376.

Blanchard, E. B., Appelbaum, K. A., Radnitz, C. L., Jaccard, J., & Dentinger, M. P. (1989). The refractory headache patient—I, Chronic, daily, high intensity headache. *Behaviour Research and Therapy, 27,* 403–410.

Blanchard, E. B., Appelbaum, K. A., Radnitz, C. L., Michultka, D., Morrill, B., Kirsch, C., Hillhouse, J., Evans, D. D., Guarnieri, P., Attanasio, V., Andrasik, F., Jaccard, J., & Dentinger, M. P. (1990). Placebo-controlled evaluation of abbreviated progressive muscle relaxation and of relaxation combined with cognitive therapy in the treatment of tension headache. *Journal of Consulting and Clinical Psychology, 58,* 210–215.

Blanchard, E. B., Appelbaum, K. A., Radnitz, C. L., Morrill, B., Michultka, D., Kirsch, C., Guarnieri, P., Hillhouse, J., Evans, D. D., Jaccard, J., & Barron, K. D. (1990). A controlled evaluation of thermal biofeedback and thermal biofeedback combined with cognitive therapy in the treatment of vascular headache. *Journal of Consulting and Clinical Psychology, 58,* 216–224.

Blanchard, E. B., Hillhouse, J., Appelbaum, K. A., & Jaccard, J. (1987). What is an adequate length of baseline in research and clinical practice with chronic headache? *Biofeedback and Self-Regulation, 12,* 323–329.

Blanchard, E. B., Kirsch, C. A., Appelbaum, K. A., & Jaccard, J. (1989). The role of psychopathology in chronic headache: Cause or effect? *Headache, 29,* 295–301.

Blanchard, E. B., Nicholson, N. L., Taylor, A. E., Steffek, B. D., Radnitz, C. L., & Appelbaum, K. A. (1991). The role of regular home practice in the relaxation treatment of tension headache. *Journal of Consulting and Clinical Psychology, 59,* 467–470.

Blanchard, E. B., O'Keefe, D., Neff, D., Jurish, S., & Andrasik, F. (1981). Interdisciplinary agreement in the diagnosis of headache types. *Journal of Behavioral Assessment, 3,* 5–9.

Blanchard, E. B., Radnitz, C. L., Evans, D. D., Schwarz, S. P., Neff, D. F., & Gerardi, M. A. (1986). Psychological comparisons of irritable bowel syndrome to chronic tension and migraine headache and nonpatient controls. *Biofeedback and Self-Regulation, 11,* 221–230.

Blanchard, E. B., Steffek, B. D., Jaccard, J., & Nicholson, N. L. (1991). Psychological changes accompanying non-pharmacological treatment of chronic headache: The effects of outcome. *Headache, 31,* 249–253.

Blanchard, E. B., Theobald, D. E., Williamson, D. A., Silver, B. V., & Brown, D. A. (1978). Temperature biofeedback in the treatment of migraine headaches. *Archives of General Psychiatry, 35,* 581–588.

Blaszczynski, A. P. (1984). Personality factors in classical migraine and tension headache. *Headache, 24,* 238–244.

Blau, J. N., & Cumings, J. N. (1966). Method of precipitating and preventing some migraine attacks. *British Medical Journal, 2,* 1242–1243.

Blau, J. N., & Dexter, S. L. (1981). The site of pain origin during migraine attacks. *Cephalalgia, 1,* 143–147.

Blau, J. N., & Diamond, S. (1985). Dietary factors in migraine precipitation: The physicians' view. *Headache, 25,* 184–187.

Blau, J. N., & Thavapalan, M. (1988). Preventing migraine: A study of precipitating factors. *Headache, 28,* 481–483.

Blumenthal, J. A., Williams, R. B. Jr., Kong, Y. H., Schonberg, S. M., & Thompson, L. W. (1978). Type A behavior patterns and coronary atherosclerosis. *Circulation, 58,* 634–639.

Bond, M. R., & Pilowsky, I. (1966). Subjective assessment of pain and its relationship to the administration of analgesics in patients with advanced cancer. *Journal of Psychosomatic Research, 10,* 203.

Borgeat, F., Hade, B., Elie, R., & Larouche, L. M. (1984). Effects of voluntary muscle tension increases in tension headache. *Headache, 24,* 199–202.

Boudewyns, P. A. (1982). Assessment of headache. In F. J. Keefe & J. A. Blumenthal (Eds.), *Assessment strategies in behavioral medicine* (pp. 167–180). New York: Grune & Stratton.

Bowdler, I., Kilian, J., & Gansslen-Blumberg, S. (1988). The association between analgesic abuse and headache—coincidental or causal? *Headache, 28,* 494.

Bradley, L. A., Prokop, C. K., Margolis, R., & Gentry, W. D. (1978). Multivariate analyses of the MMPI profiles of low back pain patients. *Journal of Behavioral Medicine, 1,* 253–272.

Breslau, N. (1992). Migraine, suicidal ideation, and suicide attempts. *Neurology, 42,* 392–395.

Breslau, N., Davis, G. C., & Andreski, P. (1991). Migraine, psychiatric disorders, and suicide attempts: An epidemiologic study of young adults. *Psychiatry Research, 37,* 11–23.

Brewerton, T. D., & George, M. S. (1990). A study of the seasonal variation of migraine. *Headache, 30,* 511–513.

Budzynski, T. H., Stoyva, J. M., Adler, C. S., & Mullaney, D. J. (1973). EMG biofeedback and tension headaches: A controlled outcome study. *Psychosomatic Medicine, 35,* 484–496.

Burns, D. D. (1980). *Feeling good: The new mood therapy.* New York: New American Library.

Callaghan, N. (1968). The migraine syndrome in pregnancy. *Neurology, 18,* 197–201.

Carlsson, J., Augustinsson, L., Blomstrand, C., & Sullivan, M. (1990). Health status in patients with tension headache treated with acupuncture or physiotherapy. *Headache, 30,* 593–599.

Carroll, J. D. (1971). Migraine: General management. *British Medical Journal, 2,* 756–757.

Chancellor, A. M., Wroe, S. J., & Cull, R. E. (1990). Migraine occurring for the first time in pregnancy. *Headache, 30,* 224–227.

Chesney, M. A., & Shelton, J. L. (1976). A comparison of muscle relaxation and electromyogram biofeedback treatments for muscle contraction headache. *Journal of Behavior Therapy and Experimental Psychiatry, 7,* 221–225.

Christiansen, V. (1925). Rapport sur la migraine. *Revue Neurologie, 32,* 855–881.

Clark, D. M. (1989). Anxiety states: Panic and generalized anxiety. In K. Hawton, P. M. Salkovskis, J. Kirk, & D. M. Clark (Eds.), *Cognitive behaviour therapy for psychiatric problems: A practical guide* (pp. 52–96). Oxford, England: Oxford University Press.

Clark, D. M., & Beck, A. T. (1988). Cognitive approaches. In C. Last & M. Hersen (Eds.), *Handbook of anxiety disorders* (pp. 71–90). Hillsdale, NJ: Erlbaum.

Cohen, M. J., McArthur, D. L., & Rickles, W. H. (1980). Comparison of four biofeedback treatments for migraine headache: Physiological and headache variables. *Psychosomatic Medicine, 42,* 463–480.

Cohen, M. J., Rickles, W. H., & McArthur, D. L. (1978). Evidence for physiological response stereotypy in migraine headache. *Psychosomatic Medicine, 40,* 344–354.

Cohen, R. A., Williamson, D. A., Monguillot, J. E., Hutchinson, P. C., Gottlieb, J., & Waters, W. F. (1983). Psychophysiological response patterns in vascular and muscle contraction headaches. *Journal of Behavioral Medicine, 6,* 93–107.

Cohen, S., Kamark, T., & Mermelstein, R. (1983). A global measure of perceived stress. *Journal of Health and Social Behavior, 24,* 385–396.

Cohen, S., Mermelstein, R., Kamarck, T., & Hoberman, H. M. (1985). Measuring the functional components of social support. In I. G. Sarason & B. R. Sarason (Eds.), *Social support: Theory, research and applications* (pp. 73–94). The Hague, Netherlands: Martinus Nijhoff.

Coles, M. G. H., Donchin, E., & Porges, S. W. (Eds.). (1986). *Psychophysiology: Systems, processes and applications.* New York: Guilford Press.

Collet, L., Cottraux, J., & Juenet, C. (1986). Tension headaches: Relation between MMPI paranoia score and pain and between MMPI hypochondriasis score and frontalis EMG. *Headache, 26,* 365–368.

242   References

Collins, F. L., & Thompson, J. K. (1979). Reliability and standardization in the assessment of self-reported headache pain. *Journal of Behavioral Assessment, 1*, 73–86.

Cox, D. J., Freundlich, A., & Meyer, R. G. (1975). Differential effectiveness of electromyograph feedback, verbal relaxation instructions, and medication placebo with tension headaches. *Journal of Consulting and Clinical Psychology, 43*, 892–898.

Cox, D. J., & Thomas, D. (1981). Relationship between headaches and depression. *Headache, 21*, 261–263.

Dalessio, D. J. (1972). *Wolff's headache and other head pain*. New York: Oxford University Press.

Dalessio, D. J. (1974). Mechanisms and biochemistry of headache. *Postgraduate Medicine, 56*, 55–62.

Dalessio, D. J., Kunzel, M., Sternbach, R., & Sovak, M. (1979). Conditioned adaptation-relaxation reflex in migraine therapy. *Journal American Medical Assocation, 242*, 2102–2104.

Dalsgaard-Nielsen, T. (1965). Migraine and heredity. *Acta Neurologica Scandinavia, 41*, 287–300.

Dalton, K. (1973). Migraine in general practice. *Journal of the Royal College of General Practitioners, 23*, 97–106.

Dalton, K. (1975). Food intake prior to a migraine attack: Study of 2,313 spontaneous attacks. *Headache, 15*, 188–193.

Daly, E. J., Donn, P. A., Galliher, J. J., & Zimmerman, J. S. (1983). Biofeedback applications to migraine and tension headaches: A double-blinded outcome study. *Biofeedback and Self-Regulation, 8*, 135–152.

Dangel, R. F., & Polster, R. A. (1988). *Teaching child management skills*. New York: Pergamon Press.

Davidson, P. (1987). Hypnosis and migraine headache: Reporting a clinical series. *Australian Journal of Clinical and Experimental Hypnosis, 15*, 111–118.

De Bedetittis, G., & Lorenzetti, A. (in press). The role of stressful life events in the persistence of primary headaches: Major events vs. daily hassles. *Pain*.

DeLozier, J. E., & Gagnon, R. O. (1975). *National ambulatory medical case survey: 1973 Summary, United States, May 1973–April 1974* (DHEW Publication No. HRA 76-1772). Washington, DC: U.S. Government Printing Office.

Demjen, S., Bakal, D. A., & Dunn, B. E. (1990). Cognitive correlates of headache intensity and duration. *Headache, 30*, 423–427.

Deubner, D. C. (1977). An epidemiologic study of migraine and headache in 10–20-year-olds. *Headache, 17*, 173–180.

Devoto, M., Lozito, A., Staffa, G., D'Alessandro, R., Sacquegna, T., & Romeo, G. (1986). Segregation analysis of migraine in 128 families. *Cephalalgia, 6*, 101–105.

Diamond, S. (1979). Headache. *American Academy of Family Physicians*, 6–21.

Diamond, S., Medina, J., Diamond-Falk, J., & DeVeno, T. (1979). The value of biofeedback in the treatment of chronic headaches: A five-year retrospective study. *Headache, 19*, 90–96.

Dieter, J. N., & Swerdlow, B. (1988). A replicative investigation of the reliability of the MMPI in the classification of chronic headaches. *Headache, 28*, 212–222.

Domino, J. V., & Haber, J. D. (1987). Prior physical and sexual abuse in women with chronic headache: Clinical correlates. *Headache, 27*, 310–314.

Downey, J. A., & Frewin, D. B. (1972). Vascular responses in the hands of patients suffering from migraine. *Journal of Neurology, Neurosurgery and Psychiatry, 35*, 258–263.

Drummond, P. D. (1982). Extracranial and cardiovascular reactivity in migrainous subjects. *Journal of Psychosomatic Research, 26*, 317–331.

Drummond, P. D. (1985). Predisposing, precipitating and relieving factors in different categories of headache. *Headache, 25*, 16–22.

Drummond, P. D. (1986). A quantitative assessment of photophobia in migraine and tension headache. *Headache, 26,* 465–469.

Drummond, P. D. (1987). Scalp tenderness and sensitivity to pain in migraine and tension headache. *Headache, 27,* 45–50.

Drummond, P. D., & Lance, J. W. (1983). Extracranial vascular changes and the source of pain in migraine headache. *Annals of Neurology, 13,* 32–37.

Drummond, P. D., & Lance, J. W. (1984). Clinical diagnosis and computer analysis of headache symptoms. *Journal of Neurology, Neurosurgery and Psychiatry, 47,* 128–133.

Dubbert, P. M., Martin, J. E., & Epstein, L. H. (1986). In K. A. Holroyd & T. L. Creer (Eds.), *Self-management of chronic disease: Handbook of clinical interventions and research* (pp. 127–161). Orlando, FL: Academic Press.

Dunkel-Schetter, C., Folkman, S., & Lazarus, R. S. (1987). Social support received in stressful situations. *Journal of Personality and Social Psychology, 53,* 71–80.

Ehde, D. M., & Holm, J. E. (1992). Stress and headache: Comparisons of migraine, tension, and headache-free subjects. *Headache Quarterly, 3,* 54–60.

Ehde, D.M., Holm, J. E., & Metzger, D. L. (1991). The role of family structure, functioning, and pain modeling in headache. *Headache, 31,* 35–40.

Ekbom, K., Ahlborg, B., & Schele, R. (1978). Prevalence of migraine and cluster headache in Swedish men of 18. *Headache, 18,* 9–19.

Elliot, K., Frewin, D. B., & Downey, J. A. (1973). Reflex vasomotor responses in hands of patients suffering from migraine. *Headache, 13,* 188–196.

Elmore, A. M., & Turksy, B. (1981). A comparison of two psychophysiological approaches to the treatment of migraine. *Headache, 21,* 93–101.

Epstein, L. H., & Abel, G. G. (1977). An analysis of biofeedback training effects for tension headache patients. *Behavior Therapy, 8,* 37–47.

Epstein, L. H., Hersen, M., & Hemphill, D. P. (1974). Music feedback in the treatment of tension headache: An experimental case study. *Journal of Behavior Therapy and Experimental Psychiatry, 5,* 59–63.

Epstein, M. T., Hockaday, J. M., & Hockaday, T. D. R. (1975). Migraine and reproductive hormones throughout the menstrual cycle. *Lancet, 1,* 543–548.

Falkenstein, M., & Hoormann, J. (1987). Psychophysiological correlates of vasomotor self-control mediated by biofeedback. *Journal of Psychophysiology, 4,* 383–392.

Falloon, I. R. H. (Ed.). (1988). *Handbook of behavioural family therapy.* London: Hutchinson.

Featherstone, H. J. (1985). Medical diagnoses and problems in individuals with recurrent idiopathic headaches. *Headache, 25,* 136–140.

Featherstone, H. J., & Beitman, B. D. (1984). Marital migraine: A refractory daily headache. *Psychosomatics, 25,* 30–38.

Fennell, M. J. V. (1989). Depression. In K. Hawton, P. M. Salkovskis, J. Kirk, & D. M. Clark (Eds.), *Cognitive behaviour therapy for psychiatric problems: A practical guide* (pp. 169–234). Oxford, England: Oxford University Press.

Fernandez, E. (1986). A classification system of cognitive coping strategies for pain. *Pain, 26,* 141–151.

Feuerstein, M. (1989). Definitions of pain. In Tollison, C. D. (Ed.), *Handbook of chronic pain management* (pp. 2–5). Baltimore, MD: Williams & Wilkins.

Feuerstein, M., Adams, H. E., & Beiman, I. (1976). Cephalic vasomotor and electromyographic feedback in the treatment of combined muscle contraction and migraine headaches in a geriatric case. *Headache, 16,* 232–237.

Feuerstein, M., Bush, C., & Corbisiero, R. (1982). Stress and chronic headache: A psychophysiological analysis of mechanisms. *Journal of Psychosomatic Research, 26,* 167–182.

Figueroa, J. L. (1982). Group treatment of chronic tension headaches. *Behavior Modification, 6,* 229–239.

Fin, T., DiGiuseppe, R., & Culver, C. (1991). The effectiveness of rational–emotive therapy in the reduction of muscle contraction headaches. *Journal of Cognitive Psychotherapy, 15,* 93–103.

Fisher, C. M. (1988). Analgesic rebound headache refuted. *Headache, 28,* 666.

Flor, H., Kerns, R. D., & Turk, D. C. (1987). The role of spouse reinforcement, perceived pain, and activity levels of chronic pain patients. *Journal of Psychosomatic Research, 31,* 251–259.

Flor, H., & Turk, D. C. (1989). Psychophysiology of chronic pain: Do chronic pain patients exhibit symptom-specific psychophysiological responses? *Psychological Bulletin, 105,* 215–259.

Fordyce, W. E. (1976). *Behavioral methods for chronic pain and illness.* St. Louis, MO: C. V. Mosby.

Fordyce, W. E., Fowler, R. S., Lehmann, J. F., DeLateur, B. J., Sand, P. L., & Trieschmann, R. B. (1973). Operant conditioning in the treatment of chronic pain. *Archives Physical Medicine Rehabilitation, 54,* 399–408.

Fowler, R. S. (1975). Operant therapy for headaches. *Headache, 15,* 63–68.

Freemon, F. R. (1968). Computer diagnosis of headache. *Headache, 8,* 49–56.

French, E. G., Lassers, B. W., & Desai, M. G. (1967). Vasomotor responses in the hands of migrainous subjects. *Journal of Neurology, Neurosurgery and Psychiatry, 30,* 276–278.

Friar, L. R., & Beatty, J. (1976). Migraine: Management by trained control of vasoconstriction. *Journal of Consulting and Clinical Psychology, 44,* 46–53.

Friedman, H. S., & Booth-Kewley, S. (1987). The "disease-prone personality": A meta-analytic view of the construct. *American Psychologist, 42,* 539–555.

Gannon, L. R., Haynes, S. N., Cuevas, J., & Chavez, R. (1987). Psychophysiological correlates of induced headaches. *Journal of Behavioral Medicine, 10,* 411–423.

Gannon, L. R., Haynes, S. N., Safranek, R., & Hamilton, J. A. (1981). A psychophysiological investigation of muscle-contraction and migraine headache. *Journal of Psychosomatic Research, 25,* 271–280.

Gatchel, R. J., Deckel, A. W., Weinberg, N., & Smith, J. E. (1985). The utility of the Milton Behavioral Health Inventory in the study of chronic headaches. *Headache, 25,* 49–54.

Gauthier, J. G., Bois, R., Allaire, D., & Drolet, M. (1981). Evaluation of skin temperature biofeedback training at two different sites for migraine. *Journal of Behavioral Medicine, 4,* 407–419.

Gauthier, J. G., Doyon, J., Lacroix, R., & Drolet, M. (1983). Blood volume pulse biofeedback in the treatment of migraine headache: A controlled evaluation. *Biofeedback and Self-Regulation, 8,* 427–442.

Gauthier, J. G., Fournier, A., & Roberge, C. (1991). The differential effects of biofeedback in the treatment of menstrual and nonmenstrual migraine. *Headache, 31,* 82–90.

Gauthier, J. G., Fradet, C., & Roberge, C. (1988). The differential effects of biofeedback in the treatment of classical and common migraine. *Headache, 28,* 39–46.

Gauthier, J. G., Lacroix, R., Cote, A., Doyon, J., & Drolet, M. (1985). Biofeedback control of migraine headaches: A comparison of two approaches. *Biofeedback and Self-Regulation, 10,* 139–159.

Goldfried, M. R., & Davison, G. (1976). *Clinical behavior therapy.* New York: Holt, Rinehart & Winston.

Goldfried, M. R., & Trier, C. (1974). Effectiveness of relaxation as an active coping skill. *Journal of Abnormal Psychology, 83,* 348–355.

Good, P. A., Taylor, R. H., & Mortimer, M. J. (1991). The use of tinted glasses in childhood migraine. *Headache, 31,* 533–536.

Goodell, H., Lewontin, R., & Wolff, H. G. (1954). Familial occurrence of migraine headache. A.M.A. *Archives of Neurology and Psychiatry, 72,* 325–335.

Gottlieb, B. H. (1988). Support interventions: A typology and agenda for research. In S. W. Duck (Ed.), *Handbook of personal relationships: Theory, research and interventions* (pp. 519–541). Chichester, England: Wiley.

Graham, J. R., & Wolff, H. G. (1938). Mechanism of migraine headache and action of ergotamine tartrate. *Archives of Neurology and Psychiatry, 39,* 737–763.

Grant, E. C. G. (1979). Food allergies and migraine. *Lancet, 1,* 966–969.

Grazzi, L., Frediani, F., Zappacosta, B., Boiardi, A., & Bussone, G. (1988). Psychological assessment in tension headache before and after biofeedback treatment. *Headache, 28,* 337–338.

Grimm, L., Douglas, D., & Hanson, P. (19871). Aerobic training in prophylaxis of migraine. *Medical Science Sports Exercise, 13,* 98.

Haber, J. D., Kuczmierczyk, A. R., & Adams, H. E. (1985). Tension headaches: Muscle overactivity or psychogenic pain. *Headache, 25,* 23–29.

Hage, P. (1981). Exercise may reduce frequency of migraine. *Physician and Sports Medicine, 9,* 24–25.

Hammen, C., & Mayol, A. (1982). Depression and cognitive characteristics of stressful life-event types. *Journal of Abnormal Psychology, 91,* 165–174.

Hanson, R. W., & Gerber, K. E. (1990). *Coping with chronic pain: A guide to patient self-management.* New York: Guilford Press.

Harrigan, J. A., Kues, J. R., Ricks, D. F., & Smith, R. (1984). Moods that predict coming migraine headaches. *Pain, 20,* 385–396.

Harrison, R. H. (1975). Psychological testing in headache: A review. *Headache, 14,* 177–185.

Harvey, P. G., & Hay, K. M. (1984). Mood and migraine—A preliminary prospective study. *Headache, 24,* 225–228.

Hatch, J. P., Prihoda, T. J., Moore, P. J., & Cyr-Provost, M. (1991). A naturalistic study of the relationship among electromyographic activity, psychological stress, and pain in ambulatory tension-type headache patients and headache-free controls. *Psychosomatic Medicine, 53,* 576–584.

Hatch, J. P., Schoenfeld, L. S., Boutros, N. N., Seleshi, E., Moore, P. J., & Cyr-Provost, M. (1991). Anger and hostility in tension-type headache. *Headache, 31,* 302–304.

Hawton, K., & Kirk, J. (1989). Problem-solving. In K. Hawton, P. M. Salkovskis, J. Kirk, & D. M. Clark (Eds.), *Cognitive behaviour therapy for psychiatric problems: A practical guide* (pp. 406–426). Oxford, England: Oxford University Press.

Haynes, S. G., Feinleib, M., & Kannel, W. B. (1980). The relationship of psychosocial factors to coronary heart disease in the Framingham study: III. Eight-year incidence of coronary heart disease. *American Journal of Epidemiology, 111,* 37–58.

Haynes, S. G., Levine, S., Scotch, N., Feinleib, M., & Kannel, W. B. (1978). The relationship of psychosocial factors to coronary heart disease in the Framingham study: I. Methods and risk factors. *American Journal of Epidemiology, 107,* 362–383.

Haynes, S. N. (1981). Muscle contraction headache: A psychophysiological perspective of etiology and treatment. In S. N. Haynes & L. R. Gannon (Eds.), *Psychosomatic disorders; A psychophysiological approach to etiology and treatment* (pp. 231–276). New York: Praeger Press.

Haynes, S. N., & Cuevas, J. L. (1980). Symptom substitution and biofeedback treatment of migraine headache: A comment. *Headache, 20,* 347–348.

Haynes, S. N., Cuevas, J., & Gannon, L. R. (1982). The psychophysiological etiology of muscle contraction headache. *Headache, 22,* 122–132.

Haynes, S. N., Falkin, S., & Sexton-Radek, K. (1989). Psychophysiological assessment in behavior therapy. In G. Turpin (Ed.), *Handbook of clinical psychophysiology* (pp. 175–214). Chichester, England: Wiley.

Haynes, S. N., Gannon, L. R., Bank, J., Shelton, D., & Goodwin, J. (1990). Cephalic blood flow correlates of induced headaches. *Journal of Behavioral Medicine, 13,* 467–480.

Haynes, S. N., Gannon, L. R., Cuevas, J., Heiser, P., Hamilton, J., & Katranides, M. (1983). The psychophysiological assessment of muscle contraction headache subjects during headache and non-headache conditions. *Psychophysiology, 20,* 393–399.

Haynes, S. N., Griffin, P., Mooney, D., & Parise, M. (1975). Electromyographic biofeedback and relaxation instructions in the treatment of muscle contraction headaches. *Behavior Therapy, 6,* 672–678.

Haynes, S. N., & O'Brien, W. H. (1990). Functional analysis in behavior therapy. *Clinical Psychology Review, 10,* 649–668.

Headache Classification Committee of the International Headache Society. (1988). Classification and diagnostic criteria for headache disorders, cranial neuralgias and facial pain. *Cephalalgia,* 8(suppl. 7), 9–96.

Heide, F. J., & Borkovec, T. D. (1983). Relaxation-induced anxiety: Paradoxical anxiety enhancement due to relaxation training. *Journal of Consulting and Clinical Psychology, 51,* 171–182.

Heide, F. J., & Borkovec, T. D. (1984). Relaxation-induced anxiety: Mechanisms and theoretical implications. *Behaviour Research and Therapy, 22,* 1–12.

Henderson, S., Byrne, D. G., & Duncan-Jones, P. (1981). *Neurosis and the social environment.* Sydney, Australia: Academic Press.

Henderson, S., Duncan-Jones, P., Byrne, D. G., & Scott, R. (1980). Measuring social relationships. The interview schedule for social interaction. *Psychological Medicine, 10,* 723–734.

Henryk-Gutt, R., & Rees, W. L. (1973). Psychological aspects of migraine. *Journal of Psychosomatic Research, 17,* 141–153.

Hering, R., & Rose, F. C. (1992). Menstrual migraine. *Headache Quarterly, 3,* 27–31.

Heyneman, N. E., Fremouw, W. J., Gano, D., Kirkland, F., & Heiden, L. (1990). Individual differences and the effectiveness of different coping strategies for pain. *Cognitive Therapy and Research, 14,* 63–77.

Hicks, R. A., & Campbell, J. (1983). Type A-B behavior and self estimates of the frequency of headaches in college students. *Psychological Reports, 52,* 912.

Hillhouse, J. J., Blanchard, E. B., Appelbaum, K. A., & Kirsch, C. (1988). The role of Type A behaviour pattern in chronic headache. *Behaviour Change, 5,* 3–8.

Hockaday, J. M., Macmillan, A. L., & Whitty, C. W. M. (1967). Vasomotor reflex response in idiopathic and hormone dependent migraine. *Lancet, 1,* 1023–1026.

Holm, J. E., Holroyd, K. A., Hursey, K. G., & Penzien, D. B. (1986). The role of stress in recurrent tension headache. *Headache, 26,* 160–167.

Holmes, T. H., & Rahe, R. H. (1967). The Social Readjustment Rating Scale. *Journal of Psychosomatic Research, 11,* 213–218.

Holroyd, K. A., & Andrasik, F. (1978). Coping and the self-control of chronic tension headache. *Journal of Consulting and Clinical Psychology, 46,* 1036–1045.

Holroyd, K. A., & Andrasik, F. (1982). A cognitive–behavioral approach to recurrent tension and migraine headache. In P. C. Kendall (Ed.), *Advances in Cognitive–Behavioral Research and Therapy* (Vol. 1, pp. 275–320). New York: Academic Press.

Holroyd, K. A., Andrasik, F., & Noble, J. (1980). A comparison of EMG biofeedback and a credible pseudotherapy in treating tension headache. *Journal of Behavioral Medicine, 3,* 29–39.

Holroyd, K. A., Andrasik, F., & Westbrook, T. (1977). Cognitive control of tension headache. *Cognitive Therapy and Research, 1,* 121–133.

Holroyd, K. A., Holm, J. R., Hursey, K. G., Penzien, D. B., Cordingley, G. E., Theofanous, A. G., Richardson, S. C., & Tobin, D. L. (1988). Recurrent vascular headache: Home-based behavioral treatment versus abortive pharmacological treatment. *Journal of Consulting and Clinical Psychology, 56,* 218–223.

Holroyd, K. A., Holm, J. F., Penzien, D. B., Cordingley, G. E., Hursey, K. G., Martin, N. J., & Theofanous, A. (1989). Long-term maintenance of improvements achieved with abortive pharmacological and nonpharmacological treatments for migraine: Preliminary findings. *Biofeedback and Self-Regulation*, 14, 301–308.

Holroyd, K. A., Nash, J. M., Pingel, J. D., Cordingley, G. E., & Jerome, A. (1991). A comparison of pharmacological (amitriptyline HCL) and nonpharmacological (cognitive–behavioral) therapies for chronic tension headaches. *Journal of Consulting and Clinical Psychology*, 59, 387–393.

Holroyd, K. A., & Penzien, D. B. (1986). Client variables and the behavioral treatment of recurrent tension headache: A meta-analytic review. *Journal of Behavioral Medicine*, 9, 515–536.

Holroyd, K. A., & Penzien, D. B. (1990). Pharmacological versus nonpharmacological prophylaxis of recurrent migraine headache: A meta-analytic review of clinical trials. *Pain*, 42, 1–13.

Holroyd, K. A., Penzien, D. B., Hursey, K. G., Tobin, D. L., Rogers, L., Holm, J. E., Marcille, P. J., Hall, J. R., & Chila, A. G. (1984). Change mechanisms in EMG biofeedback training: Cognitive changes underlying improvements in tension headache. *Journal of Consulting and Clinical Psychology*, 52, 1039–1053.

Howarth, E. (1965). Headache, personality and stress. *British Journal of Psychiatry*, 111, 1193–1197.

Hudzinski, L. G., & Lawrence, G. S. (1988). Significance of EMG surface electrode placement models and headache findings. *Headache*, 28, 30–35.

Hundleby, J. D., & Loucks, A. D. (1985). Personality characteristics of young adult migraineurs. *Journal of Personality Assessment*, 49, 497–500.

Hunt, S. M., McEwen, J., & McKenna, S. P. (1986). *Measuring health status*. London: Croom Helm.

Hursey, K. G., & Jacks, S. D. (1992). Fear of pain in recurrent headache sufferers. *Headache*, 32, 283–286.

Hutchings, D. F., & Reinking, R. H. (1976). Tension headaches: What form of therapy is most effective? *Biofeedback and Self-Regulation*, 1, 183–190.

Invernizzi, G., Gala, C., & Sacchetti, E. (1985). Life events and headache. *Cephalalgia* (Suppl. 2), 229–231.

Iversen, H. K., Langemark, M., Andersson, P. G., Hansen, P. E., & Olesen, J. (1990). Clinical characteristics of migraine and episodic tension-type headache in relation to old and new diagnostic criteria. *Headache*, 30, 514–519.

Jacob, R. G., Turner, S. M., Szekely, B. C., & Eidelman, B. H. (1983). Predicting outcome of relaxation therapy in headaches: The role of "depression." *Behavior Therapy*, 14, 457–465.

Jacobson, E. (1938). *Progressive relaxation*. Chicago: University of Chicago Press.

Jacobson, N. S., & Gurman, A. S. (Eds.). (1986). *Clinical handbook of marital therapy*. New York: Guilford Press.

Jahanshahi, M., Hunter, M., & Philips, C. (1986). The headache scale: an examination of its reliability and validity. *Headache*, 26, 76–82.

Janssen, K. (1983). Differential effectiveness of EMG feedback versus combined EMG-feedback and relaxation instructions in the treatment of tension headache. *Journal of Psychosomatic Research*, 27, 243–253.

Janssen, K., & Neutgens, J. (1986). Autogenic training and progressive relaxation in the treatment of three kinds of headache. *Behaviour Research and Therapy*, 24, 199–208.

Jenkinson, C. (1990). Health status and mood state in a migraine sample. *International Journal of Social Psychiatry*, 36, 42–48.

Jenkinson, C., & Fitzpatrick, R. (1990). Measurement of health status in patients with chronic illness: Comparison of the Nottingham Health Profile and the general health questionnaire. *Family Practice, 7*, 121–124.

Jennings, J. R., Tahmoush, A. J., & Redmond, D. P. (1980). Non-invasive measurement of peripheral vascular activity. In I. Martin & P. H. Venables (Eds.), *Techniques in psychophysiology* (pp. 69–137). Chichester, England: Wiley.

Joffe, R., Bakal, D. A., & Kaganov, J. (1983). A self-observation study of headache symptoms in children. *Headache, 23*, 20–25.

Johansson, J., & Ost, L. (1987). Temperature–biofeedback treatment of migraine headache: Special effects and the effects of "generalization training." *Behavior Modification, 11*, 182–199.

Johnson, P. R., & Thorn, B. E. (1989). Cognitive–behavioral treatment of chronic headache: Group versus individual treatment format. *Headache, 29*, 358–365.

Johnson, W. G., & Turin, A. (1975). Biofeedback treatment of migraine headache: A systematic case study. *Behavior Therapy, 6*, 394–397.

Johnston, D. W., & Martin, P. R. (1991). Psychophysiological contributions to behavior therapy. In P. R. Martin (Ed.), *Handbook of behavior therapy and psychological science: An integrative approach* (pp. 383–409). New York: Pergamon Press.

Jurish, S. E., Blanchard, E. B., Andrasik, F., Teders, J. J., Neff, D. F., & Arena, J. G., (1983). Home-versus clinic-based treatment of vascular headache. *Journal of Consulting and Clinical Psychology, 51*, 743–751.

Kabela, E., Blanchard, E. B., Appelbaum, K. A., & Nicholson, N. (1989). Self-regulatory treatment of headache in the elderly. *Biofeedback and Self-Regulation, 14*, 219–228.

Kanner, A. D., Coyne, J. C., Schaefer, C., & Lazarus, R. S. (1981). Comparison of two modes of stress measurement: Daily hassles and uplifts versus major life events. *Journal of Behavioral Medicine, 4*, 1–29.

Kashiwagi, T., McClure, J. N., & Wetzel, R. D. (1972). Headache and psychiatric disorders. *Diseases Nervous System, 33*, 659–663.

Keefe, F. J., & Dolan, E. (1986). Pain behavior and pain coping strategies in low back pain and myofascial pain dysfunction syndrome patients. *Pain, 24*, 49–56.

Kewman, D., & Roberts, A. H. (1980). Skin temperature biofeedback and migraine headaches. *Biofeedback and Self-Regulation, 5*, 327–345.

Kim, M., & Blanchard, E. B. (1992). Two studies of the nonpharmacological treatment of menstrually related migraine headaches. *Headache, 32*, 197–202.

Knapp, T. W. (1982). Evidence for sympathetic deactivation by temporal vasoconstriction and digital vasodilation biofeedback in migraine patients: A reply to Elmore and Tursky and a new hypothesis. *Headache, 22*, 233–236.

Knapp, T. W., & Florin, I. (1981). The treatment of migraine headache by training in vasoconstriction of the temporal artery and a cognitive stress-coping training. *Behavioral Analysis and Modification, 4*, 267–274.

Kneebone, I. I., & Martin, P. R. (1992). Partner involvement in the treatment of chronic headaches. *Behaviour Change, 9*, 201–215.

Koehler, S. M., & Glaros, A. (1988). The effect of aspartame on migraine headache. *Headache, 28*, 10–13.

Kohlenberg, R. J., & Cahn, T. (1981). Self-help treatment for migraine headaches: A controlled outcome study. *Headache, 21*, 196–200.

Kohler, T., & Haimerl, C. (1990). Daily stress as a trigger of migraine attacks: Results of thirteen single-subject studies. *Journal of Consulting and Clinical Psychology, 58*, 870–872.

Kondo, C., & Canter, A. (1977). True and false electromyographic feedback: Effect on tension headache. *Journal of Abnormal Psychology, 86*, 93–95.

Kremsdorf, R. B., Kochanowicz, N. A., & Costell, S. (1981). Cognitive skills training versus EMG biofeedback in the treatment of tension headaches. *Biofeedback and Self-Regulation, 6*, 93–102.

Kroner-Herwig, B., Diergarten, K., Diergarten, D., & Seeger-Siewert, R. (1988). Psychophysiological reactivity of migraine sufferers in conditions of stress and relaxation. *Journal of Psychosomatic Research, 32,* 483–492.

Kudrow, L. (1975). The relationship of headache frequency to hormone use in migraine. *Headache, 15,* 36–40.

Kudrow, L. (1978). Current aspects of migraine headache. *Psychosomatics, 19,* 48–57.

Kudrow, L., & Sutkus, B. J. (1979). MMPI pattern specificity in primary headache disorders. *Headache, 19,* 18–24.

Kunzer, M. B. (1987). Marital adjustment of headache: Sufferers and their spouses. *Journal of Psychosocial Nursing, 25,* 13–17.

L'Abate, L., & Milan, M. A. (Eds.). (1985). *Handbook of social skills training and research.* New York: Wiley.

Lacey, J. M., Kagen, J., Lacey, B. C., & Moss, H. A. (1962). The visceral level: Situational determinants and behavioral correlates of autonomic response patterns. In P. Knapp (Ed.), *Expression of emotions in men.* New York: International University Press.

Lacroix, R., & Barbaree, H. E. (1990). The impact of recurrent headaches on behavior lifestyle and health. *Behaviour Research and Therapy, 28,* 235–242.

Lai, C., Dean, P., Ziegler, D. K., & Hassanein, R. S. (1989). Clinical and electrophysiological responses to dietary challenge in migraineurs. *Headache, 29,* 180–186.

Lake, A. E. (1981). Behavioral assessment considerations in the management of headache. *Headache, 21,* 170–178.

Lake, A. E., Rainey, J., & Papsdorf, J. D. (1979). Biofeedback and rational–emotive therapy in the management of migraine headache. *Journal of Applied Behavior Analysis, 12,* 127–140.

Lance, F., Parkes, C., & Wilkinson, M. (1988). Does analgesic abuse cause headache de novo? *Headache, 28,* 61–62.

Lance, J. W. (1973). *The mechanism and management of headache* (2nd ed.). London: Butterworths.

Lange, A. J., & Jakubowski, P. (1976). *Responsible assertive behavior: Cognitive/behavioral procedures for trainers.* Champaign, IL: Research Press.

Largen, J. W., Mathew, R. J., Dobbins, K., & Claghorn, J. L. (1981). Specific and nonspecific effects of skin temperature control in migraine management. *Headache, 21,* 36–44.

Lazarus, R. S., & Folkman, S. (1984). *Stress, appraisal and coping.* New York: Springer.

Lehrer, P. M., & Murphy, A. I. (1991). Stress reactivity and perception of pain among tension headache sufferers. *Behaviour Research and Therapy, 29,* 61–69.

Lethem, J., Slade, P. D., Troup, J. D. G., & Bentley, G. (1983). Outline of a fear–avoidance model of exaggerated pain perception—I. *Behaviour Research and Therapy, 21,* 401–408.

Levine, B. A. (1984). Effects of depression and headache type on biofeedback for muscle-contraction headaches. *Behavioural Psychotherapy, 12,* 300–307.

Leviton, A. (1984). To what extent does food sensitivity contribute to headache recurrence? *Developmental Medicine and Child Neurology, 26,* 539–545.

Leviton, A., Slack, M. V., Masek, B., Bana, D., & Graham, J. R. (1984). A computerized behavioral assessment for children with headaches. *Headache, 24,* 182–185.

Levor, R. M., Cohen, M. J., Naliboff, B. D., McArthur, D., & Heuser, G. (1986). Psychosocial precursors and correlates of migraine headache. *Journal of Consulting and Clinical Psychology, 54,* 347–353.

Levy, L. M. (1983). An epidemiological study of headache in an urban population in Zimbabwe. *Headache, 23,* 2–9.

Lichstein, K. L., Fischer, S. M., Eakin, T. L., Amberson, J. I., Bertorini, T., & Hoon, P. W. (1991). Psychophysiological parameters of migraine and muscle-contraction headaches. *Headache, 31,* 27–34.

Lisspers, J., & Ost, L. (1990a). BVP biofeedback in the treatment of migraine: The effects of constriction and dilatation during different phases of the migraine attack. *Behavior Modification, 14*, 200–221.

Lisspers, J., & Ost, L. (1990b). Long-term follow-up of migraine treatment: Do the effects remain up to six years? *Behaviour Research and Therapy, 28*, 313–322.

Lockett, D. C., & Campbell, J. F. (1992). The effects of aerobic exercise on migraine. *Headache, 32*, 50–54.

Lucas, R. N. (1977). Migraine in twins. *Journal of Psychosomatic Research, 20*, 147–156.

MacLeod, C., & Mathews, A. M. (1991). Cognitive–experimental approaches to the emotional disorders. In P. R. Martin (Ed.), *Handbook of behavior therapy and psychological science: An intergrative approach* (pp. 116–150). New York: Pergamon Press.

Marcus, D. A., & Soso, M. J. (1989). Migraine and stripe-induced visual discomfort. *Archives of Neurology, 46*, 1129–1132.

Marrelli, A., Marini, C., & Prencipe, M. (1988). Seasonal and meterological factors in primary headaches. *Headache, 28*, 111–113.

Martin, I., & Venables, P. H. (1980). *Techniques in psychophysiology.* Chichester, England: Wiley.

Martin, M. J. (1966). Tension headache, a psychiatric study. *Headache, 6*, 47–54.

Martin, M. J. (1972). Muscle-contraction headache. *Psychosomatics, 13*, 16–19.

Martin, M. J. (1983). Muscle-contraction (tension) headache. *Psychosomatics, 24*, 319–324.

Martin, P. R. (1983). Behavioural research on headaches: Current status and future directions. In K. A. Holroyd, B. Schlote, & H. Zenz (Eds.), *Perspectives in research on headache* (pp. 204–215). Lewiston, NY: Hogrefe.

Martin, P. R. (1985). Classification of headache: The need for a radical revision. *Cephalalgia, 5*, 1–4.

Martin, P. R. (1986). Headaches. In N. J. King & A. Remenyi (Eds.), *Health care: A behavioural approach* (pp. 145–157). Sydney, Australia: Grune & Stratton.

Martin, P. R., Marie, G. V., & Nathan, P. R. (1987). Behavioral research on headaches: A coded bibliography. *Headache, 27*, 555–570.

Martin, P. R., Marie, G. V., & Nathan, P. R. (1992). Psychophysiological mechanisms of chronic headaches: Investigation using pain induction and pain reduction procedures. *Journal of Psychosomatic Reseaerch, 36*, 132–148.

Martin, P. R., & Mathews, A. M. (1978). Tension headaches: Psychophysiological investigation and treatment. *Journal of Psychosomatic Research, 22*, 389–399.

Martin, P. R., Milech, D., & Nathan, P. R. (1992). *Towards a functional model of chronic headaches: Investigation of antecedents and consequences.* Manuscript submitted for publication.

Martin, P. R., & Nathan, P. R. (1987). Differential prevalence rates for headaches: A function of stress and social support? *Headache, 27*, 329–333.

Martin, P. R., Nathan, P. R., & Milech, D. (1987). The Type A behaviour pattern and chronic headaches. *Behaviour change, 4*, 33–39.

Martin, P. R., Nathan, P. R., Milech, D., & van Keppel, M. (1988). The relationship between headaches and mood. *Behaviour Research and Therapy, 26*, 353–356.

Martin, P. R., Nathan, P. R., Milech, D., & van Keppel, M. (1989). Cognitive therapy vs. self-management training in the treatment of chronic headaches. *British Journal of Clinical Psychology, 28*, 347–361.

Martin, P. R., Rose, M. J., Nichols, P. J. R., Russell, P., & Hughes, I. (19860) Physiotherapy exercises for low back pain: Process and clinical outcome. *International Rehabilitation Medicine, 8*, 34–38.

Martin, P. R., & Soon, K. (1992). *The relationship between perceived stress, social support and chronic headache.* Manuscript submitted for publication.

Martin, P. R., & Theunissen, C. (1992). *The role of life event stress, coping and social support in chronic headaches*. Manuscript submitted for publication.

Mathew, N. T., Kurman, R., & Perez, F. (1990). Drug-induced refractory headache: Clinical features and management. *Headache, 30,* 634–638.

Mazzella, C. (1992). *Chocolate as a precipitant of headache.* Unpublished master's thesis, University of Western Australia, Perth, Australia.

McAnulty, D. P., Rappaport, N. B., Waggoner, C. D., Brantley, P. J., Barkemeyer, C., & McKenzie, S. J. (1986). Psychopathology in volunteers for headache research: Initial versus later respondents. *Headache, 26,* 37–38.

McCaffery, M. (1979). *Nursing management of the patient with pain* (2nd ed.). Philadelphia: J. B. Lippincott.

McCaffrey, R. J., Goetsch, V. L., Robinson, J., & Isaac, W. (1986). Differential responsivity of the vasomotor response system to a "novel" stressor. *Headache, 26,* 240–242.

McFall, R. M. (1970). The effects of self-monitoring on normal smoking behavior. *Journal of Consulting and Clinical Psychology, 35,* 135–142.

McKay, M., & Fanning, P. (1987). *Self-esteem.* Oakland, CA: New Harbinger.

McNair, D. M., & Lorr, M. (1982). *Profile of Mood States—Bipolar Form (POMS-Bi).* Educational and Industrial Testing Service, San Diego, CA.

Medina, J. L., & Diamond, S. (1978). The role of diet in migraine. *Headache, 18,* 31–34.

Meichenbaum, D. H. (1975). A self-instructional approach to stress management: A proposal for stress inoculation training. In C. D. Spielberger & I. G. Sarason (Eds.), *Stress and anxiety* (Vol. 1, pp. 237–263). New York: Wiley.

Meichenbaum, D. H. (1977). *Cognitive–behavior modification: An integrative approach.* New York: Plenum Press.

Melzack, R. (1975). The McGill Pain Questionnaire: Major properties and scoring methods. *Pain, 1,* 277–299.

Melzack, R. (1983). The McGill Pain Questionnaire. In R. Melzack (Ed.), *Pain measurement and assessment* (pp. 412–47). New York: Raven Press.

Melzack, R., & Wall, P. D. (1988). *The challenge of pain* (rev. ed.). London: Penguin.

Merskey, H. (1972). Personality traits of psychiatric patients with pain. *Journal of Psychosomatic Research, 16,* 163.

Merskey, H. (Ed.). (1986). Classification of chronic pain: Descriptions of chronic pain syndromes and definitions of pain terms. *Pain* (suppl. 3), S1–S225.

Michultka, D. M., Blanchard, E. B., Appelbaum, K. A., Jaccard, J., & Dentinger, M. P. (1989). The refractory headache patient—II. High medication consumption (analgesic rebound) headache. *Behaviour Research and Therapy, 27,* 411–420.

Mindell, J. A., & Andrasik, F. (1987). Headache classification and factor analysis with a pediatric population. *Headache, 27,* 96–101.

Mitchell, K. R., & Mitchell, D. M. (1971). Migraine: An exploratory treatment application of programmed behaviour therapy techniques. *Journal of Psychosomatic Research, 15,* 137–157.

Mitchell, K. R., & White, R. G. (1977). Behavioral self-management: An application to the problem of migraine headaches. *Behavior Therapy, 8,* 213–221.

Mizener, D., Thomas, M., & Billings, R. (1988). Cognitive changes of migraineurs receiving biofeedback training. *Headache, 28,* 339–343.

Moffett, A. M., Swash, M., & Scott, D. F. (1974). Effect of chocolate in migraine: A double-blind study. *Journal of Neurology, Neurosurgery and Psychiatry, 37,* 445–448.

Monks, R., & Taenzer, P. (1983). A Comprehensive Pain Questionnaire. In R. Melzack (Ed.), *Pain measurement and assessment* (pp. 233–237). New York: Raven Press.

Morley, S. (1977). Migraine: A generalized vasomotor dysfunction? A critical review of evidence. *Headache, 17,* 71–74.

Morley, S. (1985). An experimental investigation of some assumptions underpinning psychological treatments of migraine. *Behaviour Research and Therap;y*, 23, 65–74.

Morrill, B., & Blanchard, E. B. (1989). Two studies of the potential mechanisms of action in the
thermal biofeedback treatment of vascular headache. *Headache*, 29, 169–176.

Morrison, D. P., & Price, W. H. (1989). The prevalence of psychiatric disorder among female
new referrals to a migraine clinic. *Psychological Medicine*, 19, 919–925.

Mosley, T. H., Penzien, D. B., Johnson, C. A., Brantley, P. J., Wittrock, D. A., Andrew, M.
E., & Payne, T. J. (1990, November). *Stress and headache: A time-series approach.* Paper
presented at the 24th meeting of the Association for Advancement of Behavior Therapy,
San Francisco, CA.

Mullinix, J. M., Norton, B. J., Hack, S., & Fishman, M. A. (1978). Skin temperature
biofeedback and migraine. *Headache*, 17, 242–244.

Murphy, A. I., & Lehrer, P. M. (1990). Headache versus nonheadache state: A study of
electrophysiological and affective changes during muscle contraction headaches. *Behavioral Medicine*, 16, 23–29.

Murphy, A. I., Lehrer, P. M., & Jurish, S. (1990). Cognitive coping skills and relaxation
training as treatments for tension headaches. *Behavior Therapy*, 21, 89–98.

Newland, C. A., Illis, L. S., Robinson, P. K., Batchelor, B. G., & Waters, W. E. (1978). A
survey of headache in an English city. *Research Clinical Studies in Headache*, 5, 1–20.

Newton, C. R., & Barbaree, H. E. (1987). Cognitive changes accompanying headache treatment: The use of a thought-sampling procedure. *Cognitive Therapy and Research*, 11,
635–652.

Nikiforow, R., & Hokkanen, E. (1978). An epidemiological study of headache in an urban and
rural population in Northern Finland. *Headache*, 18, 137–145.

Norton, G. R., & Nielson, W. R. (1977). Headaches: The importance of consequent events.
Behavior Therapy, 8, 504–506.

Novaco, R. W. (1979). The cognitive regulation of anger and stress. In P. C. Kendall & S. D.
Hollon (Eds.), *Cognitive–behavioral interventions: Theory, research and procedures* (pp.
241–285). New York: Academic Press.

O'Banion, D. R. (1981). Dietary control of headache pain, five case studies. *Journal of Holistic
Medicine*, 3, 140–151.

O'Brien, M. D. (1971). Cerebral blood changes in migraine. *Headache*, 10, 139–143.

Ostfeld, A. M., & Wolff, H. G. (1958). Identification, mechanisms and management of the
migraine syndrome. *Medical Clinics of North America*, 42, 1497–1509.

Otis, L. S., Turner, A., & Low, D. (1975). *EMG training and headache reduction: Some
methodological issues.* Paper presented at Biofeedback Society Meeting, Monterey, CA.

Packard, R. C., Andrasik, F., & Weaver, R. (1989). When headaches are good. *Headache*, 29,
100–102.

Parry, G. (1988). Mobilizing social support. In F. N. Watts (Ed.), *New developments in clinical
psychology* (Vol. 2, pp. 83–104). Chichester, England: Wiley/British Psychological Society.

Passchier, J., Schouten, J., van der Donk, J., & van Romunde, L. K. J. (1991). The association
of frequent headaches with personality and life events. *Headache*, 31, 116–121.

Passchier, J., van der Helm-Hylkema, H., & Orlebeke, J. F. (1984a). Psychophysiological
characteristics of migraine and tension headache patients. Differential effects of sex and
pain state. *Headache*, 24, 131–139.

Passchier, J., van der Helm-Hylkema, H., & Orlebeke, J. F. (1984b). Personality and headache
type: A controlled study. *Headache*, 24, 140–146.

Paulin, J. M., Waal-Manning, H. S., Simpson, F. O., & Knight, R. G. (1985). The prevalence
of headache in a small New Zealand town. *Headache*, 25, 147–151.

Paykel, E. S., Prusoff, B. A., & Uhlnhuth, E. H. (1971). Scaling of life events. *Archives of
General Psychiatry*, 25, 340–347.

Payne, T. J., & Colletti, G. (1991). Treatment of a 15-year-old girl with chronic muscle-contraction headache using implosive therapy. *British Journal of Medical Psychology, 64*, 173–177.

Payne, T. J., Stetson, B., Stevens, V. M., Johnson, C. A., Penzien, D. B., & van Dorsten, B. (1991). The impact of cigarette smoking on headache activity in headache patients. *Headache, 31*, 329–332.

Pearce, S. (1983). A review of cognitive–behavioral methods for the treatment of chronic pain. *Journal of Psychosomatic Research, 27*, 431–440.

Peck, C. L., & Kraft, G. H. (1977). Electromyographic biofeedback for pain related to muscle tension. *Archives of Surgery, 112*, 889–895.

Peck, D. F., & Attfield, M. E. (1981). Migraine symptoms on the Waters Headache Questionnaire: A statistical analysis. *Journal of Psychosomatic Research, 25*, 281–288.

Penzien, D. B., Holroyd, K. A., Holm, J. E., & Hursey, K. G. (1985). Psychometric characteristics of the Bakal Headache Assessment Questionnaire. *Headache, 25*, 55–58.

Penzien, D. B., Johnson, C., Carpenter, D., & Holroyd, K. (1990). Drug vs. behavioral treatment of migraine: Long-acting propranol vs. home-based self-management training. *Headache, 30*, 300.

Peterson, R. A. (1991). Psychosocial determinants of disorder: Social support, coping and social skills interactions. In P. R. Martin (Ed.), *Handbook of behavior therapy and psychological science: An integrative approach* (pp. 270–282). New York: Pergamon Press.

Phanthumchinda, K., & Sithi-Amorn, C. (1989). Prevalence and clinical features of migraine: A community survey in Bangkok, Thailand. *Headache, 29*, 594–597.

Philips, H. C. (1976). Headache and personality. *Journal of Psychosomatic Research, 20*, 535–542.

Philips, H. C. (1977a). Headache in general practice. *Headache, 16*, 322–329.

Philips, H. C. (1977b). A psychological analysis of tension headache. In S. Rachman (Ed.), *Contributions to medical psychology* (Vol. 1, pp. 91–131), Oxford, England: Pergamon Press.

Philips, H. C. (1977c). The modification of tension headache pain using EMG biofeedback. *Behaviour Research and Therapy, 15*, 119–129.

Philips, H. C. (1987a). Avoidance behaviour and its role in sustaining chronic pain. *Behaviour Research and Therapy, 25*, 273–279.

Philips, H. C. (1987b). The effects of behavioural treatment on chronic pain. *Behaviour Research and Therapy, 25*, 365–377.

Philips, H. C. (1988). *The psychological management of chronic pain: A treatment manual.* New York: Springer.

Philips, H. C., & Hunter, M. (1981). Pain behavior in headache sufferers. *Behavior Analysis and Modification, 4*, 257–266.

Philips, H. C., & Hunter, M. S. (1982a). A psychophysiological investigation of tension headache. *Headache, 22*, 173–179.

Philips, H. C., & Hunter, M. (1982b, January). Headache in a psychiatric population. *Journal of Nervous and Mental Disease, 170*, 34–41.

Philips, H. C., & Jahanshahi, M. (1985). Chronic pain: An experimental analysis of the effects of exposure. *Behaviour Research and Therapy, 23*, 281–290.

Philips, H. C., & Jahanshahi, M. (1986). The components of pain behaviour report. *Behaviour Research and Therapy, 24*, 117–125.

Poppen, R. (1988). *Behavioral relaxation training and assessment.* New York: Pergamon Press.

Poppen, R., & Maurer, J. (1982). Electromyographic analysis of relaxed postures. *Biofeedback and Self-Regulation, 7*, 491–498.

Pozniak-Patewicz, E. (1976). "Cephalgic" spasm of head and neck muscles. *Headache, 16*, 261–266.

Price, K. P., & Blackwell, S. (1980). Trait levels of anxiety and psychological responses to stress in migraineurs and normal controls. *Journal of Clinical Psychology*, 36, 658–660.

Raczynski, J. M., & Thompson, J. K. (1983). Methodological guidelines for clincal headache research. *Pain*, 15, 1–18.

Raczynski, J. M., Ray, W. J., & McCarthy, P. (1991). Psychophysiological assessment. In M. Hersen, A. E. Kazdin, & A. S. Bellack (Eds.), *The clinical psychology handbook* (2nd ed., pp. 465–490). New York: Pergamon Press.

Radnitz, C. L., Appelbaum, K. A., Blanchard, E. B., Elliott, L., & Andrasik, F. (1988). The effect of self-regulatory treatment on pain behavior in chronic headache. *Behaviour Research and Therapy*, 26, 253–260.

Radnitz, C. L., Blanchard, E. B., & Bylina, J. (1990). A preliminary report of dietary therapy as a treatment for refraction migraine headache. *Headache Quarterly*, 1, 239–343.

Ramsden, R., Friedman, B., & Williamson, D. (1983). Treatment of childhood headache reports with contingency management procedures. *Journal of Clinical Child Psychology*, 12, 202–206.

Rapoport, A. M. (1988). Analgesic rebound headache. *Headache*, 28, 662–665.

Rapoport, A. M. (1992). The diagnosis of migraine and tension-type headache, then and now. *Neurology*, 42(suppl. 2), 11–15.

Rapoport, A. M., Weeks, R. E., Sheftell, F. D., Baskin, S. M., & Verdi, J. (1985). Analgesic rebound headache: Theoretical and practical implications. *Cephalalgia*, 5(suppl. 3), 448–449.

Rappaport, N. B., McAnulty, D. P., & Brantley, P. J. (1988). Exploration of the Type A behavior pattern in chronic headache sufferers. *Journal of Consulting and Clinical Psychology*, 56, 621–623.

Rappaport, N. B., McAnulty, D. P., Waggoner, C. D., & Brantley, P. J. (1987). Cluster analysis of Minnesota Multiphasic Personality Inventory (MMPI) profiles in a chronic headache population. *Journal of Behavioral Medicine*, 10, 49–60.

Raskin, N. H. (1988). *Headache* (2nd ed.). New York: Churchill Livingstone.

Rasmussen, B. K., Jensen, R., & Olesen, J. (1991). Questionnaire versus clinical interview in the diagnosis of headache. *Headache*, 31, 290–295.

Reading, C. (1984). Psychophysiological reactivity in migraine following biofeedback. *Headache*, 24, 70–74.

Reading, C., & Mohr, P. D. (1976). Biofeedback control of migraine: A pilot study. *British Journal of Social and Clinical Psychology*, 15, 429–433.

Reinking, R. H., & Hutchings, D. (1981). Follow-up to: "Tension headaches: What form of therapy is most effective?" *Biofeedback and Self-Regulation*, 6, 57–62.

Review Panel. (1981). Coronary-prone behavior and coronary heart disease: A critical review. *Circulation*, 63, 1199–1215.

Richardson, G. M., & McGrath, P. J. (1989). Cognitive–behavioral therapy for migraine headaches: A minimal-therapist-contact approach versus a clinic-based approach. *Headache*, 29, 352–357.

Richey, E. T., Kooi, K. A., & Waggoner, R. W. (1966). Visually evoked responses in migraine. *Electroencephalography Clinical Neurophysiology*, 21, 23–27.

Rimm, D. C., & Masters, J. C. (1979). *Behavior therapy: Techniques and empirical findings* (2nd ed.). New York: Academic Press.

Robinson, M. E., Geisser, M. E., Dieter, J. N., & Swerdlow, B. (1991). The relationship between MMPI cluster membership and diagnostic category in headache patients. *Headache*, 31, 111–115.

Rojahn, J., & Gerhards, F. (1986). Subjective stress sensitivity and physiological responses to an aversive auditory stimulus in migraine and control subjects. *Journal of Behavioral Medicine*, 9, 203–212.

Roskies, E. (1983). Stress management for Type A individuals. In D. Meichenbaum & M. E. Jaremko (Eds.), *Stress reduction and prevention* (pp. 261–288). New York: Plenum Press.

Rowsell, A. R., Neylan, C., & Wilkinson, M. (1973). Ergotamine-induced headaches in migrainous patients. *Headache, 13*, 65–67.

Roy, R. (1986). Marital conflicts and exacerbation of headache: Some clinical observations. *Headache, 26*, 360–364.

Roy, R. (1989). Couple therapy and chronic headache: A preliminary outcome study. *Headache, 29*, 455–457.

Ryan, R. E. (1954). *Headache: Diagnosis and treatment.* St. Louis, MO: C. V. Mosby.

Rybstein-Blinchik, E. (1979). Effects of different cognitive strategies on chronic pain experience. *Journal of Behavioral Medicine, 2*, 93–101.

Sachs, H., Sevilla, F., Barberis, P., Bolis, L., Schoenberg, B., & Cruz, M. (1985). Headache in the rural village of Quiroga, Ecuador. *Headache, 25*, 190–193.

Salkovskis, P. M. (1989). Somatic problems. In K. Hawton, P. M. Salkovskis, J. Kirk, & D. M. Clark (Eds.), *Cognitive behaviour therapy for psychiatric problems: A practical guide* (pp. 235–276). Oxford, England: University Press.

Saper, J. R. (1978). Miagraine: II. treatment. *Journal American Medical Association, 239*, 2480–2484.

Saper, J. R. (1987). Ergotamine dependency: A review. *Headache, 27*, 435–438.

Saper, J. R. (1989). Chronic headache syndromes. *Neurologic Clinics, 7*, 387–411.

Sarason, I. G., Levine, H. M., Basham, R. B., & Sarason, B. R. (1983). Assessing social support: The Social Support Questionnaire. *Journal of Personality and Social Psychology, 44*, 127–139.

Sargent, J. D., Green, E. E., & Walters, E. D. (1972). The use of autogenic feedback training in a pilot study of migraine and tension headaches. *Headache, 12*, 120–124.

Sargent, J. D., Green, E. E., & Walters, E. D. (1973). Preliminary report on the use of autogenic feedback training in the treatment of migraine and tension headaches. *Psychosomatic Medicine, 35*, 129–135.

Sargent, J. D., Solbach, P., Coyne, L., Spohn, H., & Segerson, J. (1986). Results of a controlled, experimental, outcome study of nondrug treatments for the control of migraine headaches. *Journal of Behavioral Medicine, 9*, 291–323.

Sargent, J. D., Walters, E. D., & Green, E. E. (1973). Psychosomatic self-regulation of migraine headaches. *Seminars in Psychiatry, 5*, 415–428.

Sauber, W. J. (1980). What is Chinese restaurant syndrome? *Lancet, 1*, 721–722.

Schilling, D. J., & Poppen, R. (1983). Behavioral relaxation training and assessment. *Journal of Behavior Therapy and Experimental Psychiatry, 14*, 99–107.

Schlutter, L. C., Golden, C. J., & Blume, H. G. (1980). A comparison of treatments for prefrontal muscle contraction headache. *British Journal of Medical Psychology, 53*, 47–52.

Schmidt, F. N., Carney, P., & Fitzsimmons, G. (1986). An empirical assessment of the migraine personality type. *Journal of Psychosomatic Research, 30*, 189–197.

Schoenen, J., Bottin, D., Hardy, F., & Gerard, P. (1991). Cephalic and extracephalic pressure thresholds in chronic tension-type headache. *Pain, 47*, 145–149.

Schultz, J. H., & Luthe, W. (1959). *Autogenic training: A psychophysiologic approach in psychotherapy.* New York: Grune & Stratton.

Schultz, J. H., & Luthe, W. (1969). *Autogenic therapy* (Vols. I–VI). New York: Grune & Stratton.

Scopp, A. L. (1991). MSG and hydrolyzed vegetable protein induced headache: Review and case studies. *Headache, 31*, 107–110.

Scott, D. S. (1979). A comprehensive treatment strategy for muscle contraction headaches. *Journal of Behavior Therapy and Experimental Psychiatry, 10*, 35–40.

Selby, G., & Lance, J. W. (1960). Observations on 500 cases of migraine and allied vascular headache. *Journal of Neurology, Neurosurgery and Psychiatry, 23,* 23–32.

Sherman, R. A. (1982). Home use of tape-recorded relaxation exercises as initial treatment for stress related disorders. *Military Medicine, 147,* 1062–1066.

Sillanpaa, M. (1976). Prevalence of migraine and other headache in Finnish children starting school. *Headache, 16,* 288–290.

Sillanpaa, M. (1983). Changes in the prevalence of migraine and other headaches during the first seven school years. *Headache, 23,* 15–19.

Simone, S., & Long, M. (1985). Marital cognitive–behavioral treatment for chronic tension headache: A case study. *Behavior Therapist, 8, 26,* 36–37.

Skinhoj, E., & Paulson, O. B. (1969). Regional blood flow in internal carotid distribution during migraine attack. *British Medical Journal, 3,* 569–570.

Slade, P. D., Troup, J. D. G., Lethem, J., & Bentley, G. (1983). The fear–avoidance model of exaggerated pain perception II: Preliminary studies of coping strategies for pain. *Behaviour Research and Therapy, 21,* 409–416.

Sokolov, E. N. (1963). *Perception and the conditioned reflex.* New York: Pergamon Press.

Solbach, P., Sargent, J. D., & Coyne, L. (1984). Menstrual migraine headache: Results of a controlled, experimental, outcome study of non-drug treatments. *Headache, 24,* 75–78.

Solbach, P., Sargent, J. D., & Coyne, L. (1989). An analysis of home practice for non-drug headache treatments. *Headache, 29,* 528–531.

Sorbi, M., & Tellegen, B. (1986). Differential effects of training in relaxation and stress-coping in patients with migraine. *Headache, 26,* 473–481.

Sorbi, M., & Tellegen, B. (1988). Stress-coping in migraine. *Social Science in Medicine, 26,* 351–358.

Sorbi, M., Tellegen, B., & Du Long, A. (1989). Long-term effects of training in relaxation and stress-coping in patients with migraine: A 3-year follow-up. *Headache, 29,* 111–121.

Sovak, M., Kunzel, M., Sternbach, R. A., & Dalessio, D. J. (1981). Mechanism of the biofeedback therapy of migraine: Volitional manipulation of the psychophysiological background. *Headache, 21,* 89–92.

Spanier, G. B. (1976). Measuring dyadic adjustment: New scales for assessing the quality of marriage and similar dyads. *Journal of Marriage and the Family, 38,* 15–28.

Spanos, N. P., Horton, C., & Chaves, J. F. (1975). The effect of two cognitive strategies on pain threshold. *Journal of Abnormal Psychology, 84,* 677–681.

Spielberger, C. D., Gorsuch, R. L., & Lushene, R. G. (1970). *The state-trait anxiety inventory.* Palo Alto, CA: Consulting Psychologists Press.

Steger, J. C., & Harper, R. G. (1980). Comprehensive biofeedback versus self-monitored relaxation in the treatment of tension headache. *Headache, 20,* 137–142.

Steptoe, A. (1991). Psychobiological processes in the etiology of disease. In P. R. Martin (Ed.), *Handbook of behavior therapy and psychological science: An integrative approach* (pp. 325–347). New York: Pergamon Press.

Sternbach, R. A. (1974). *Pain patients: Traits and treatment.* New York: Academic Press.

Sternbach, R. A., Dalessio, D. J., Kunzel, M., & Bowman, G. E. (1980). MMPI patterns in common headache disorders. *Headache, 20,* 311–315.

Sternbach, R. A., & Timmermans, G. (1975). Personality change associated with reduction of pain. *Pain, 1,* 177–181.

Stout, M. A. (1984). A cognitive–behavioral study of self-reported stress factors in migraine headache. *Psychopathology, 17,* 290–296.

Stout, M. A. (1985). Homeostatic reconditioning in stress-related disorders: A preliminary study of migraine headaches. *Psychotherapy, 22,* 531–541.

Sturgis, E. T., & Arena, J. G. (1984). Psychophysiological assessment. *Progress in Behavior Modification, 17,* 1–30.

Sturgis, E. T., Tollison, C. D., & Adams, H. E. (1978). Modification of combined migraine-muscle contraction headaches using BVP and EMG feedback. *Journal of Applied Behavior Analysis, 11*, 215–223.

Szajnberg, N., & Diamond, S. (1980). Biofeedback, migraine headache and new symptom formation. *Headache, 20*, 29–31.

Szekely, B., Botwin, D., Eidelman, B. H., Becker, M., Elman, N., & Schemm, R. (1986). Nonpharmacological treatment of menstrual headache: Relaxation–biofeedback behavior therapy and person-centered insight therapy. *Headache, 26*, 86–92.

Takeshima, T., & Takahashi, K. (1988). The relationship between muscle contraction headache and migraine: A multivariate analysis study. *Headache, 28*, 272–277.

Tan, S.-Y. (1982). Cognitive and cognitive–behavioral methods for pain control: A selective review. *Pain, 12*, 201–228.

Taylor, J. A. (1953). A personality scale of manifest anxiety. *Journal of Abnormal and Social Psychology, 48*, 285–290.

Teders, S. J., Blanchard, E. B., Andrasik, F., Jurish, S. E., Neff, D. F., & Arena, J. G. (1984). Relaxation training for tension headache: Comparative efficacy and cost-effectiveness of a minimal therapist contact versus a therapist delivered procedure. *Behavior Therapy, 15*, 59–70.

Theorell, T. (1989). Personal control at work and health: A review of epidemiological studies in Sweden. In A. Steptoe & A. Appels (Eds.), *Stress, personal control and health* (pp. 49–64). Chichester, England: Wiley.

Thompson, J. K., & Collins, F. L. (1979). Reliability of headache questionnaire data. *Headache, 19*, 97–101.

Thompson, J. K., & Figueroa, J. L. (1980). Dichotomous vs. interval rating of headache symptomatology: An investigation of the reliability of headache assessment. *Headache, 20*, 261–265.

Thompson, J. K., & Figueroa, J. L. (1983). Critical issues in the assessment of headache. *Progress in Behavior Modification, 15*, 81–111.

Tobin, D. L., Holroyd, K. A., Baker, A., Reynolds, R. V. C., & Holm, J. E. (1988). Development and clinical trial of a minimal contact, cognitive–behavioral treatment for tension headache. *Cognitive Therapy and Research, 12*, 325–339.

Toole, J. F., Brady, W. A., Cochrane, C. M., & Olmos, N. (1974). Use of computerized questionnaire in the etiologic diagnosis of headache. *Headache, 14*, 73–76.

Tunis, M. M., & Wolff, H. G. (1953). Studies on headache: Long-term observations of the reactivity of the cranial arteries in subjects with vascular headache of the migraine type. *Archives of Neurology Psychiatry, 70*, 551–557.

Turin, A., & Johnson, W. G. (1976). Biofeedback therapy for migraine headaches. *Archives of General Psychiatry, 33*, 517–519.

Turk, D. C. (1976). *An expanded skills training approach for the treatment of experimentally induced pain.* Unpublished doctoral dissertation. University of Waterloo.

Turk, D. C., & Genest, M. (1979). Regulation of pain: The application of cognitive and behavioral techniques for prevention and remediation. In P. C. Kendall & S. D. Hollon (Eds.), *Cognitive–behavioral interventions: Theory, research and practices* (pp. 287–318). New York: Academic Press.

Turk, D. C., Meichenbaum, D., & Genest, M. (1983). *Pain and behavioral medicine: A cognitive–behavioral perspective.* New York: Guilford Press.

Turkat, I. D., & Adams, H. E. (1982). Covert positive reinforcement and pain modification: A test of efficacy and theory. *Journal of Psychosomatic Research, 26*, 191–201.

Turkat, I. D., Brantley, P. J., Orton, K., & Adams, H. E. (1981). Reliability of headache diagnosis. *Journal of Behavioral Assessment, 3*, 1–4.

Turner, J. A., & Clancy, S. (1986). Strategies for coping with chronic low back pain: Relationship to pain and disability. *Pain, 24*, 355–364.

Turpin, G. (Ed.). (1989). *Handbook of clinical psychophysiology*. Chichester, England: Wiley.

Turpin, G. (1991). Psychophysiology and behavioral assessment: Is there scope for theoretical frameworks? In P. R. Martin (Ed.), *Handbook of behavior therapy and psychological science: An integrative approach* (pp. 348–382). New York: Pergamon Press.

Tursky, B. (1976). The development of a pain perception profile: A psychophysical approach. In M. Weisenberg & B. Tursky (Eds.), *Pain: New perspectives in therapy and research* (pp. 171–194). New York: Plenum Press.

Uknis, A., & Silberstein, S. D. (1991). Review article: Migraine and pregnancy. *Headache, 31*, 372–374.

van den Bergh, V., Amery, W. K., & Waelkens, J. (1987). Trigger factors in migraine: A study conducted by the Belgian migraine society. *Headache, 27*, 191–196.

Vincent, A. J. P., Spierings, E. L. H., & Messinger, H. B. (1989). A controlled study of visual symptoms and eye strain factors in chronic headache. *Headache, 29*, 523–527.

Waters, W. E. (1971). Migraine: Intelligence, social class, and familial prevalence. *British Medical Journal, 2*, 77–81.

Waters, W. E. (1973). The epidemiological enigma of migraine. *International Journal of Epidemiology, 2*, 189–194.

Waters, W. E. (1974). The Pontypridd headache survey. *Headache, 14*, 81–90.

Waters, W. E. (1978). The prevalence of migraine. *Headache, 18*, 53–54.

Watts, J. (1991). *Precipitating factors in chronic headache sufferers*. Unpublished manuscript, University of Western Australia, Perth, Australia.

Weisenberg, M. (1989). Cognitive aspects of pain. In P. D. Wall & R. Melzack (Eds.), *Textbook of pain* (2nd ed.) (pp. 231–241). Edinburgh: Churchill Livingstone.

Weiss, H. D., Stern, B. J., & Goldberg, J. (1991). Post-traumatic migraine: Chronic migraine precipitated by minor head or neck trauma. *Headache, 31*, 451–456.

Wilkins, A., Nimmo-Smith, I., Tait, A., McManus, C., Sala, S. D., Tilley, A., Arnold, K., Barrie, M., & Scott, S. (1984). A neurological basis for visual discomfort. *Brain, 107*, 989–1017.

Wilkinson, M. (1988). Treatment of migraine. *Headache, 28*, 659–661.

Williams, D. E., Thompson, J. K., Haber, J. D., & Raczynski, J. M. (1986). MMPI and headache: A special focus on differential diagnosis, prediction of treatment outcome, and patient-treatment matching. *Pain, 24*, 143–158.

Williamson, D. A., Monguillot, J. E., Jarrell, H. P., Cohen, R. A., Pratt, J. M., & Blouin, D. C. (1984). Relaxation for the treatment of headache: Controlled evaluation of two group programs. *Behavior Modification, 8*, 407–424.

Winkler, R. C. (1979). Self-management procedures for chronic headache. In K. Jonson & V. Mladenovic (Eds.), *Proceedings of the 1st Australian Conference on Behavior Modification*. New York: Auklia.

Winkler, R. C., Underwood, P., James, R., & Fatovich, B. (1982). The relative effectiveness of self-management groups and general practice in the treatment of chronic headache. In J. L. Sheppard (Ed.), *Advances in behavioural medicine* (Vol. II, pp. 255–268). Sydney, Australia: Cumberland College of Health Sciences.

Wolff, H. G. (1937). Personality features and reactions of subjects with migraine. *Archives of Neurology Psychiatry, 37*, 895–921.

Wolff, H. G., Tunis, M. M., & Goodell, H. (1953). Studies on headache: Evidence of tissue damage and changes in pain sensitivity in subjects with vascular headaches of the migraine type. *Transactions Association American Physicians, 66*, 332–341.

Wolpe, J. (1958). *Psychotherapy by reciprocal inhibition*. Stanford, CA: Stanford University Press.

Wolpe, J., & Lazarus, A. A. (1966). *Behavior therapy techniques: A guide to the treatment of neuroses*. New York: Pergamon Press.

Woods, P. J., & Burns, J. (1984). Type A behavior and illness in general. *Journal of Behavioral Medicine, 7*, 411–415.

Woods, P. J., Morgan, B. T., Day, B. W., Jefferson, T., & Harris, C. (1984). Findings on a relationship between Type A behavior and headaches. *Journal of Behavioral Medicine, 7*, 227–286.

World Health Organization. (1977). *International classification of diseases, 1975 revision.* Geneva, Switzerland, Author.

Yen, S., & McIntire, R. W. (1971). Operant therapy for constant headache complaints: A simple response–cost approach. *Psychological Reports, 28*, 267–270.

Zhao, F., Tsay, J., Cheng, X., Wong, W., Li, S., Yao, S., Chang, S., & Schoenberg, B. S. (1988). Epidemiology of migraine: A survey in 21 provinces of the People's Republic of China, 1985. *Headache, 28*, 558–565.

Ziegler, D. K. (1978). The epidemiology and genetics of migraine. *Research Clinical Studies in Headache, 5*, 21–33.

Ziegler, D. K., Hassanein, R. S., & Couch, J. R. (1977). Characteristics of life headache histories in a non-clinic population. *Neurology* (Minneapolis), *27*, 265–269.

Ziegler, D. K., Hassanein, R., & Hassanein, K. (1972). Headache syndromes suggested by factor analysis of symptom variables in a headache prone population. *Journal of Chronic Diseases, 25*, 353–363.

Zung, W. W. K. A. (1965). A self-rating depression scale. *Archives of General Psychiatry, 12*, 63–70.

Index